# SOCIAL ENTREPRENEURSHIP IN ART THERAPY



This book explores social entrepreneurship in art therapy through case studies presented by the contributing authors, highlighting the work of art therapists who have used innovative and collaborative approaches to increase access to art therapy services and promote system-level changes within the communities and institutions where they practice.

As creative changemakers, art therapists are often developing innovative solutions to address social problems impacting the communities they serve. This book reveals practical aspects of these initiatives by offering strategies, skills, and practice-based examples. By addressing issues related to equity, inclusion, and access through innovative programming, grassroots advocacy, and policy development, the authors demonstrate how their entrepreneurial initiatives in art therapy produce social impact.

Practitioners in art therapy and allied mental health professions will be inspired to seek and embrace opportunities for innovation.

**Jennifer Marie DeLucia**, DAT, ATR-BC, LCAT, is an art therapist, educator, and founding chair of the Department of Creative Arts Therapy at Syracuse University.

"If you have wondered how to bring your innovative ideas in art therapy to fruition and impact in this world, this is a must-read for you. The chapters in this book offer frameworks and successful model examples from around the world, on how art therapists can create sustainable solutions that align with the needs of the user/consumer/market. The book offers a range of new insights on how to create meaningful enterprises in art therapy that also have societal value. A primer on the personal and professional dimension of entrepreneurship, this book will help you feel energized and inspired to transform your approach for increased real-world impact."

**Girija Kaimal,** *EdD, MA, ATR-BC,*
*professor and chair of Drexel University's*
*Department of Creative Arts Therapies*
*and past president of the*
*American Art Therapy Association*

# SOCIAL ENTREPRENEURSHIP IN ART THERAPY

## CREATIVE CHANGEMAKERS IN ACTION

**Edited by Jennifer Marie DeLucia**

Routledge
Taylor & Francis Group
NEW YORK AND LONDON

Designed cover image: © Cover art created by Jennifer Marie DeLucia

First published 2026
by Routledge
605 Third Avenue, New York, NY 10158

and by Routledge
4 Park Square, Milton Park, Abingdon, Oxon, OX14 4RN

*Routledge is an imprint of the Taylor & Francis Group, an informa business*



ISBN: 978-1-032-61576-9 (hbk)
ISBN: 978-1-032-60397-1 (pbk)
ISBN: 978-1-032-61577-6 (ebk)

DOI: 10.4324/9781032615776

Typeset in New Baskerville
by Apex CoVantage, LLC

*For Sofia and Ella. You inspire me every day with your limitless creativity.*

# Contents

# Figures

# Contributors

**Mary Andrus**, DAT, LCAT, LPC, ATCS, ATR-BC (she/her), is an able-bodied, genderqueer, white woman, a mother, artist, musician, introvert, art therapist, filmmaker, and teacher. She currently co-directs the Master's in Art Therapy Program in the Graduate School of Counseling and Education at Lewis & Clark College. While working as an educator training students to become art therapists, she co-founded Art for Social Change, a group that uses meaningful art making, community building, and activism to impact people in the Portland, Oregon community. Mary specializes in treating people with trauma, integrating EMDR, IFS, Polyvagal theory, narrative, feminist, relational, and somatic approaches into her teaching and work. She has a passion for learning, hiking, creativity, and connecting with other humans.

**Chandra Davis**, ATR-BC, LCPC, LCPAT, LPC, ATCS, MIND BODY ART THERAPY LLC (she/her), is a board-certified art therapist, licensed clinical counselor, and professorial lecturer at George Washington University. With a private practice in Maryland, she infuses art therapy and archetypal psychology with internal family systems, intersectionality, and psychodynamic healing. Passionate about addressing generational trauma and fostering collective healing in black, indigenous, and people of color communities, Davis has been working in this field since 2007. Her expertise spans clinical, educational, and community-based settings, where she merges creative expression with psychological insight to support holistic well-being.

**Jennifer Marie DeLucia**, DAT, ATR-BC, LCAT, Syracuse University (she/her), is a registered, board-certified art therapist and licensed creative arts therapist (NY). She is an assistant professor and founding chair of the Department of Creative Arts Therapy at Syracuse University in Syracuse, New York. DeLucia is interested in community-based approaches to art therapy, the use of art therapy to address the needs of military-connected individuals, how art engagement in public spaces can help to promote empathy and understanding across diverse populations, and the cocreation of knowledge through participatory approaches to research, art therapy practice, and education. Her work is informed by 20 years of clinical and community-based experience in related settings.

**Rose Ehemann**, PhD, MAS, HFP, Living Museum Society Switzerland (she/her), is an art therapist, cultural manager, and founder and director of the Living Museum Wil of the Psychiatry St. Gallen and Stiftung Heimstätten Wil in Switzerland since 2002. She earned her doctorate at the University of Cologne in Germany in 2014 with research on "Virtual Reality Art Therapy." She is a guest lecturer at different universities worldwide. Her research focus is on the use of new media in art therapy and the development of the Living Museum model. From 2008 to 2012, she was president of the art therapy association in Switzerland, GPK, and has been president of the Living Museum Society Switzerland since 2012. Her interest lies in adapting the Living Museum model in different institutions worldwide by creating caring communities and networks to foster Dr. Janos Marton's vision of a "mushrooming of Living Museums all over the world."

**Emily Goldstein Nolan**, DAT, ATR-BC, LCAT, Syracuse University (she/they), is a professor of practice and practicum/internship coordinator at Syracuse University, a professional counselor, and an art therapist. In 2012, she created Bloom Art and Integrated Therapies, Inc., a community-based, nonprofit art therapy in Milwaukee, WI. Nolan develops and oversees the community art therapy programs for Bloom. She is dedicated to education and research in art therapy and working with people who have experienced trauma and oppression to feel seen, heard, and understood.

**Yasmin Henderson**, ATR-BC, LIMHP, LPC, LADC (she/her), Creative Counseling and Studio, is a board-certified registered art therapist, licensed independent mental health practitioner (Nebraska), licensed professional counselor, and licensed alcohol and drug counselor. Henderson is an entrepreneur, educator, and advocate with over two decades of experience in social services and a decade as a practicing dually licensed therapist. She assisted in the successful licensure bid in Nebraska. Henderson is the founder and owner of Creative Counseling and Studio and the founder and executive director of Inclusive Healers of the Heartland, Inc. Her work prioritizes advocacy for marginalized communities.

**Emery Hurst Mikel**, MA, ATR-BC, LCAT, LPAT, Water & Stone, Firefly & Phoenix (she/her), is the founder and director of Water & Stone, a Creative Arts Therapy PLLC, and Firefly & Phoenix LLC, both based in New York City. Water & Stone is a group practice that provides contemplative psychotherapy and creative arts therapy to the surrounding community, partners with local organizations to offer accessible services, and creates community through group support both on-site and virtually. Mikel's therapeutic specialties include working with people experiencing loss or grief and supporting women who want to build confidence and embrace their strengths. Through Firefly & Phoenix, Mikel offers professional mentoring, supervision, and continuing education courses. She is also an adjunct faculty in several graduate programs in the United States and collaborates internationally to bring workshops or trainings to therapists abroad. Mikel's goal is to build relationships focused on trust, respect, and celebrating people's inherent wisdom.

**Jennifer Jividen Jackson**, LIMHP, LPC, ATR-BC (she/her), Heartland Counseling Services, is an art therapist, mental health advocate, and nonprofit leader with over 20 years of experience. She has dedicated her career to expanding access to mental healthcare through art therapy, trauma-informed approaches, and innovative program development. Jackson played a key role in securing art therapy licensure in both Kentucky and Nebraska, advocating for the recognition of the profession and its impact on mental health treatment. She has worked in diverse settings, using creative interventions to support individuals in healing and personal growth. Her early clinical work led her to leadership roles, and she has spent the past 13 years as the Executive Director of Heartland Counseling Services, Inc., in Nebraska. Under her leadership, the organization has expanded its services to include permanent supported housing, school-based mental health programs, and crisis stabilization efforts.

**Lisa Lounsbury**, MA, LMFT, ATR-BC, Art Lab Rx, LLC (she/her), is a licensed marriage and family therapist, registered board-certified art therapist, and certified grief support specialist (Minnesota [MN]). She is the founder and executive director of Art Lab Rx, LLC, in Minneapolis, MN. Transformation is the focus of Lounsbury's business and life journey. Her past is filled with what she calls "texture," and she lights up when describing how God redeemed her. With her team, Lounsbury seeks to increase awareness of the transformational effect of art therapy. With the mobile studio, they have served the mental health needs of thousands within the state of Minnesota. She says, "This is the hardest work I've ever loved."

**Jenelle Miller**, MS, LIMHP, ATR, Open Door Mission (she/her), is a licensed independent mental health practitioner (LIMHP), registered art therapist (ATR), and published researcher. Miller's professional objective is to become a pioneer in the field of behavioral and mental health by using creative strategies and systems to promote well-being and growth in individuals and communities. With a focus on leadership and innovation, she aims to advance the field through research and practice that integrates art therapy, evidence-based therapies, and Christian ministry to develop effective and sustainable approaches to mental health treatment. Miller initiated the Nebraska Art Therapy Licensure Coalition while studying art therapy at George Washington University.

**Mitra Reyhani Ghadim**, DAT, ATR-BC, LCAT, ATCS, Living Museum NY, Pratt Institute, Long Island University (she/they), is an artist, art therapist, author, and educator. She is the director of the Living Museum of the New York State Office of Mental Health at Creedmoor Psychiatric Center and a visiting associate professor at Pratt Institute and Long Island University. She worked as a museum art therapist at the Queens Museum and Nassau County Museum of Art. She has managed museum-based programs, established community art and health services through partnership with various organizations, and published in that area. Reyhani Ghadim is interested in the application of Deleuze and Guattari's concepts of nomadism in art therapy and in the proliferation of Living Museums in disadvantaged communities globally.

**Zachary D. Van Den Berg**, MA, LPC, ATR-BC (they/he), a graduate of Adler University with an MA in Counseling: Art Therapy and a BFA from the School of the Art Institute of Chicago, has held various leadership roles within the art therapy community. At present, they are the founder and president of the 501(c)(3) nonprofit Coalition for Queer Creative Arts Therapies, Inc., and chair its annual Expressing Pride symposium. Dedicated to advancing liberatory queer and trans care practices within art therapy, they have published several peer-reviewed papers, chapters, and presentations on sexual and gender diversity and are authoring and editing a forthcoming book through Routledge Press, *Queer Worldmaking in Art Therapy: Theory & Praxis* (in press, Summer 2026). They also practice art therapy with LGBTQIA+ individuals and groups across the lifespan at Community Arts, LLC, in Austin, TX.

**Pamela Whitaker**, PhD, Belfast School of Art, Ulster University (she/her), is a lecturer in art psychotherapy. She practices under the name of Groundswell, a social enterprise dedicated to the art of gardening, creative hospitality, and festivity. She contributes to Ulster University's ethos of people, place, and partnership by producing public events that make art happen in everyday places. She has published on topics that extend art therapy into civic life—the walking studio, festival art therapy, and the nature of the commons. An advocate for ecologies of care, she co-designs art installations that gather the materials of people's lives together as an assemblage that nurtures belonging, pride of place, and the narration of life stories.

**Jessica Woolhiser Stallings**, DAT, ATR-BC, LMHP, LIMHP, LPC, Heartland Family Service (she/her), is the associate clinical director for Heartland Family Service in Nebraska and Iowa. She is a registered board-certified art therapist, licensed mental health counselor (Iowa), licensed mental health professional and counselor (Nebraska), and soon-to-be licensed art therapist (Nebraska). With 20 years of experience as an art therapist and 17 years as an art therapy educator, Stallings specializes in trauma and neurodiversity. She authored *Special Interests in Art Therapy with Autistic People: A Neurodiversity Positive Approach to Empower and Engage Participants.* As a neurodivergent (ADHD) adult, she is passionate about elevating the voices of neurodivergent clients. Stallings helped lead the successful licensure bid in NE and is an adjunct professor at the University of Nebraska Omaha, teaching future allied professionals and art therapists.

# Acknowledgments

This book was inspired by the creative and entrepreneurial colleagues I have been privileged to learn from and work with over the years. Although we often only see each other once a year at the American Art Therapy Association national conference, this annual opportunity to engage in conversations about the innovative and impactful work we are engaged in motivated me to explore our collective experiences of entrepreneurship more deeply. Thank you to the many colleagues who inspired this book, especially its 13 contributing authors.

I am grateful for the support and encouragement of Elisa Dekaney and Lynn Kapitan. Their mentorship and guidance provided a steady foundation as I worked on this book. Thank you to my department colleagues at Syracuse University: Emily Goldstein Nolan, Rochele Royster, and Bryan Bradford. I greatly value the culture of support and collaboration we have fostered. A special thank you to Girija Kaimal for reading the manuscript for this book and providing encouraging feedback.

I would also like to acknowledge the financial support from Syracuse University's Faculty Creative Activities and Research (FCAR) Grant Program, which made this research and publication possible. In addition, I am grateful to Syracuse University's College of Visual and Performing Arts for supporting and valuing my research and scholarship.

Thank you to Rudy Leon for your expertise and thoughtful editing, which significantly enhanced the quality and clarity of this book.

Finally, I want to express my deepest gratitude to my readers for your interest and support. I hope that this book inspires and resonates with you as much as it has with me.

# Introduction

## The Theory and Practice of Social Entrepreneurship

*Jennifer Marie DeLucia*

It would be a challenge to find an art therapist who has not had the experience of creating something from nothing. Creation, defined as the act of bringing something into existence, or the act of making, inventing, or producing (Merriam-Webster, 2023), is a process central to the work of art therapists across settings, populations, theoretical orientations, and art practices. At the very foundation of art therapy practice, art therapists support people as they engage with art making and the creative process to improve cognitive functions, foster self-awareness, cultivate emotional resilience, promote insight, enhance social skills, reduce and resolve conflicts, and advance societal and ecological change (American Art Therapy Association, 2017). Art therapists are often accustomed to being the sole art therapist in their organization and many have had the experience of establishing art therapy services in communities, organizations, and other settings where they had not previously existed. Social entrepreneurship is embedded in the art therapy profession and has been formally discussed through the frameworks of advocacy and social justice work (e.g., Allen, 2011; Kaplan, 2007; Talwar, 2018).

### DEFINING SOCIAL ENTREPRENEURSHIP, INTRAPRENEURSHIP, EXTRAPRENEURSHIP, AND SOCIAL INNOVATION

There is an ongoing debate within the field of social entrepreneurship about its definition and boundaries. The discourse primarily revolves around how social entrepreneurship distinguishes itself from traditional business entrepreneurship and other social initiatives. Conventionally,

DOI: 10.4324/9781032615776-1

individuals tend to associate nonprofit organizations with the creation of social value, and for-profit entities are often perceived as responsible for generating economic value. Social entrepreneurship merges these two interests by bringing social interest and market value together to create a new type of initiative that creates both social and economic value.

Nicholls' (2006) observation about the lack of consensus regarding the boundaries of social entrepreneurship is still relevant today. The definition and scope of social entrepreneurship continue to be topics of discussion in the field. Scale has been discussed as a defining boundary, with some arguing that social entrepreneurship produces major "sea-change movements" and impact (Thompson et al., 2000, p. 328). On the other hand, recognizing social entrepreneurship on a microscale is also crucial, as it acknowledges the diverse ways in which individuals and organizations can contribute to social change.

The criteria identified by Dees (2001) for determining whether the actions of an individual can be considered socially entrepreneurial provide a foundational understanding of what it means to be a social entrepreneur. Social entrepreneurs play the role of change agents in the social sector by (1) adopting a mission that is focused on creating social value; (2) recognizing and pursuing new opportunities to address social issues; (3) engaging in a process of continuous innovation, adaptation, and learning; (4) acting boldly and not being limited by resource constraints; and (5) exhibiting heightened accountability through transparent goals and outcomes.

Dees and Anderson (2006) were proponents of an inclusive or extended perspective on social entrepreneurship based on the argument that the decision about what kind of legal business to form for a venture is simply a choice about which tool to use and not a factor for considering an organization socially entrepreneurial. There are a number of characteristics that distinguish social entrepreneurs from regular entrepreneurs and traditional charities. Lepoutre et al. (2013) discussed three criteria that stand out in the literature: the predominance of a social mission, the importance of innovation, and the creation of social value. For the purposes of this book, social entrepreneurship will be considered to have three defining criteria:

(1) *Social Mission.* Social entrepreneurs have some form of explicit social objective or mission; their top priority is the creation of social value.
(2) *Innovative Approach.* Social entrepreneurship implies that an innovative solution is designed to address a complex social problem.
(3) *Sustainable Solution.* Planning for sustainability is a critical aspect of social entrepreneurship, as social challenges often require long-term commitment.

I will be referring to *social entrepreneurship* throughout this book as the process of implementing innovative and sustainable solutions to address a social or environmental issue (Short et al., 2009). Social entrepreneurs may center their efforts on identifying and addressing local social needs on a small scale. They may concentrate on filling gaps in services that impact underserved populations, introducing innovation that spans a wider social system. Or they may target systemic issues within existing social structures through large-scale revolutionary change (Zahra et al., 2009). Social entrepreneurs address income and sustainability as they relate to the various initiatives described in this book. Some produce earned income, others are grant-funded, and several are supported through coordinated volunteer efforts. To distinguish initiatives, we use the term *social enterprise* to refer to business entities that operate with the primary goal of achieving social value while also generating revenue.

Social entrepreneurship that involves existing organizations can take two forms, intra- and extra-entrepreneurship. *Social intrapreneurship,* a term used to describe some of the initiatives discussed in this book, refers to change and innovation that occurs *within* an existing organization. Social intrapreneurs contribute and implement new ideas, serve as catalysts for change, and promote changes in behavior, skills, and culture within standing organizations (Mohedano-Suanes & Benitez, 2018). *Social extrapreneurship* refers to the initiatives that work *across* organizations and institutions to mobilize the resources of several entities in new ways to address social challenges and promote social change (Chahine, 2023; Paul & Neil, 2017).

*Social innovation* is another key term used throughout the book. Social innovation is a broader concept than social entrepreneurship and refers to "innovative activities and services that are motivated by the goal of meeting a social need" (Mulgan, 2006, p. 146). Social innovation refers to the *process* of developing, implementing, and scaling new ideas that address an identified need or social issue. Social innovation can occur across a variety of settings and is a key feature of social entrepreneurship (Nandan et al., 2019).

## KEY TASKS ASSOCIATED WITH SOCIAL ENTREPRENEURSHIP

Social entrepreneurship involves several key tasks addressed in a nonlinear, iterative process that includes (1) identifying and understanding a social issue, (2) identifying interested parties and key partners, (3) conducting community-based research, (4) designing solutions, (5) developing a social business model, (6) measuring outcomes, (7) ensuring sustainability, (8) mobilizing resources and funding, (9) scaling initiatives for greater impact, (10) advocating and promoting awareness, (11) adapting and innovating to meet evolving needs, and (12) leading ethically and transparently (e.g., Chahine, 2023).

## Getting Started

The first and most crucial step in addressing a social challenge is to develop a deep understanding of the issues, grounded in data. Data are collected by conducting research into the problem and through a process of co-construction of knowledge with people who are most impacted by the problem or those with lived experience of the issue. It is important to have knowledge about how the challenge was addressed in the past, as well as an understanding of what has failed and what has been successful, and why. The full scope of this research supports social entrepreneurs in identifying and understanding the key factors contributing to the identified problem and the underlying root causes. Later, in the process, the social entrepreneur can make a determination to address one or more of the factors related to the challenge or to tackle the root causes of the problem (Chahine, 2023). Practicing cultural humility and engaging community members through participatory action research strategies and appreciative inquiry can support social entrepreneurs in effectively understanding social issues and collaborating with impacted communities on potential solutions.

### *Cultural Humility*

Lovenia Jackson (2020) stated, "social change begins with cultural humility, which is fostered in the knowing of self" (p. 117). Social entrepreneurs must have a deep awareness of their own values, beliefs, and assumptions. Cultural humility involves acknowledging and challenging one's own cultural biases, stereotypes, and assumptions and actively seeking to learn and understand others' perspectives and experiences. Practicing cultural humility can help ensure that social entrepreneurs do not impose their values and beliefs on others and inadvertently cause harm. Practicing cultural humility involves practicing self-reflection and self-critique, addressing power imbalances, and maintaining openness to understand and learn from others' perspectives and experiences.

### *Community Participation*

Community participation is a necessary component of the success of social entrepreneurship. Efforts that are not grounded in the culture or values of the community served, and efforts that do not have long-term sustainability, will fail to address the identified needs in meaningful ways, and further, may cause harm. Change prescribed by an outside party may be rejected by people who may potentially benefit from the change; they may feel imposed upon or that their voice and needs were not accurately represented in the development of the proposed solution (Bornstein & Davis, 2010). When efforts are inclusive and grounded in the culture of the community served, there are equal opportunities for members of the community to share power and resources, leading to an integration of values, beliefs, and vision across all members engaged with and impacted by the initiative (Kummitha, 2017). A rights-based approach to community participation views participation as a basic right, emphasizing the agency of people in communities to build their own lives (Kummitha, 2017).

Participatory approaches to research can help to structure participation and action. Social entrepreneurs can be viewed as action researchers, in that they learn primarily through experimentation (Bornstein & Davis, 2010). Kapitan (2018) defined action research as "a process of deconstructing knowledge to critically explore the social dimensions of practice (e.g., settings, rules, routines and habits, communication patterns, and/or uses of knowledge)" with the overall goal being change (p. 156). Participatory action research (PAR) is "collectively organized" action research that aims to transform or change a social issue. PAR involves active participation from the community impacted by the problem in all aspects of the inquiry, from defining the problem to collecting data and developing and implementing action steps (Kapitan, 2018).

The cycle of action research involves (1) collaboratively identifying the problem, (2) organizing information gathered about the problem into themes, (3) strategic action planning to address the fundamental themes identified, (4) taking action (implementing strategies), and (5) reflection-on-action—reviewing the results and consequences of the action taken. This process can occur multiple times, and some steps may be repeated to refine decisions about how to best address the identified problem. Action research supports the objectives of social entrepreneurship; community participants decide what the problem is and shape the solutions, ensuring that the initiative addresses the needs and interests of the community (Tasker et al., 2010).

### *Appreciative Inquiry*

Appreciative inquiry is a process for facilitating positive change that uses a generative approach to identifying solutions and actions within organizations (Cooperrider & Whitney, 2005). Appreciative inquiry can also be applied to work in communities, as it promotes participation and actions that emerge from within communities. The framework follows a model, called the 4 Ds, that includes (1) Discover, working together to identify strengths and core competencies; (2) Dream, collectively envisioning possibilities for the future; (3) Design, designing processes to achieve opportunities that have been identified; and (4) Destiny, detailing a collaborative path forward that commits to contributing to the strengths and supporting the achievement of the aspirations (Cooperrider & Stavros as cited in Armstrong et al., 2020). Appreciative inquiry uses generative questions to explore possibilities, approaches problems with curiosity, views problems as opportunities, and identifies strengths and successes to explore how they might be mobilized to produce the desired changes (Armstrong et al., 2020). Although originally developed as a framework for promoting positive change in organizations, appreciative inquiry can be used in other group and community settings to guide affirming processes that are inclusive and promote change rooted in the needs and experiences of those impacted.

## Planning for Sustainability

Another major area of consideration in social entrepreneurship is sustainability. Sustainability requires addressing needs in ways that are meaningful, impactful, and ethical. Initiatives that fail to address sustainability will likely fall short in addressing social issues. Social challenges are complex, multilayered, and perpetuated by structural barriers and inequalities embedded in society. Sustainability requires long-term engagement and commitment.

Community engagement involves community members in cocreating solutions and helping new initiatives to grow roots and be sustainable. Tactical strategies such as developing a business model, measuring outcomes, and mobilizing resources and funding are central to ensuring sustainability. Designing for scalability and replicability is also a consideration, as social entrepreneurs consider the long-term vision for initiatives and explore their potential to amplify impact. Planning for sustainability should be considered from the beginning and should guide how initiatives are shaped and how continuity is designed.

### *Developing a Social Business Model*

A business model describes how a company delivers value to its customers (Beugre, 2016). Business models in social entrepreneurship consider social value and sustainability and are commonly referred to in the literature as sustainability models or social business models. Social needs are often enduring, and so the social entrepreneur needs to develop a strategy that will address needs over the long term. A social business model is defined as "creating, delivering, and capturing value" for all key partners and interested parties, or anyone who will influence or is influenced by the outcome, decisions, or activities associated with a project or intervention (Beugre, 2016, p. 110). Where the business model is concerned with generating a profit, the social business model focuses on how to sustain an initiative while addressing a social problem. The Social Business Model Canvas (Table I.1) is a tool that can be used to help frame, understand, and communicate key features of the social entrepreneurial business strategy (Sparviero, 2019). This tool can help to create a shared language around a particular initiative, support brainstorming and collaboration, and serve as a foundation to ground the generation and implementation of innovative ideas with a framework centered around the social value proposition.

### *Measuring Social Outcomes*

A key component for success and sustainability in any social entrepreneurial initiative is the ability to measure and report outcomes. Outcomes are the desired changes resulting from the actions taken to address the target issue. Social entrepreneurs must determine if the changes observed would have occurred in the absence of the interventions. One way to assess this is to list all potential factors that may influence the outcome; some may be observable and not related to the intervention. Measuring social outcomes requires consideration beyond counting the number of people served; it must capture how their lives were changed as a result of the interventions (Chahine, 2023). Outputs like the number of people served can constitute valuable information to report to key partners; however, the outcomes, or broader and longer-term impacts, demonstrate the social impact of the initiative more specifically. Funders and key partners often place a higher value on outcomes and use this data to evaluate their investments and determine allocation of future support.

There are a few key things social entrepreneurs must consider when developing a measurement and evaluation plan:

1. Start early, with identifying what data will demonstrate outcomes for the initiative and then collecting that data when the project begins.
2. Embed measurement tools into existing processes, by considering ways to collect data that do not create extra work for providers or participants.
3. Choose selective measures. Consider quality over quantity when deciding how many measures are needed to demonstrate outcomes.

***Table I.1*** *Social Business Model Canvas*

| | | | | |
|---|---|---|---|---|
| **Governance**<br>What is the organizational structure that will support the initiative (e.g., governing rules, boards, or committees)? | | | | |
| *Key Partners (KPs)/ Interested Parties (IP)* | *Key Activities* | *Social Value Proposition* | *Customer and Beneficiaries Engagement* | *Customers and Beneficiaries* |
| Who are the KPs/IPs that might be impacted by the activities?<br>Who are KPs/IPs that are partners (not customers or intended beneficiaries)? | What are the most important actions or activities that need to be performed to achieve the social value proposition? | What problem will be addressed?<br>How will addressing this problem have an impact? | Who needs to be involved to ensure success? | Who do you intend to reach and serve? |
| | **Key Resources**<br>What are the most important resources needed to execute the activities?<br>How will the resources be acquired? | | **Channels**<br>How will beneficiaries be reached?<br>How will you get information to your intended audience? | |
| *Cost Structure* | | | *Income/Sustainability* | |
| What are the costs associated with the initiative (e.g., money, time, and people needed to perform the activities)?<br><br>**Intended Impact**<br>What are the intended long-term end states or goals? | | | What are the resources needed to ensure costs are covered and that the initiative has long-term sustainability (e.g., grants, donations, earned income)? | |

*Source.* Adapted from Beugre, 2016; Chahine, 2023; Sparviero, 2019.

4. Assess results with key partners and beneficiaries. Plan to share and review results with key people involved in the initiative to create feedback loops that can help to refine measurement efforts and to create pathway for using data to inform future decisions and strategies (Chahine, 2023).

### Growing Impact

Advocating and promoting awareness, adapting and innovating to meet evolving needs, and leading ethically and transparently are all ways social entrepreneurs promote sustainability and set conditions to scale the impact of a successful initiative. Once an initiative gains momentum and is producing the desired outcomes, social entrepreneurs may consider joining forces with other key partners to lobby for policy changes and resources that address the targeted challenges on a societal level (Chahine, 2023). Outcome data will support advocacy efforts to expand the reach, impact, or effectiveness of a program or intervention. Scaling initiatives involve strategies and actions designed to increase the size, scope, or sustainability of a successful initiative so that it can benefit more people or communities. Strategies for scaling impact may include replication or expansion of services or programs; partnerships and collaborations to leverage resources, share knowledge, and coordinate action; advocating for policy change; and capacity building of individuals, organizations, or communities. Collective impact and community of practice frameworks offer structure and guidance for collaborative approaches and cross-sector collaborations.

#### *Collective Impact*

Collective impact is a framework for addressing social issues through cross-sector collaboration (Hanleybrown et al., 2012). Social problems are complex in nature and methods for solving these problems are not clear and are often beyond the resources or authority of any single organization. Solutions require that key partners and interested parties examine the problem and implement interventions together, adapting their own behavior in the process (Kania & Kramer, 2011). The collective impact framework offers five pillars that guide the practice of collaboration: (1) a common agenda, (2) shared measurement systems, (3) mutually reinforcing activities, (4) continuous communication, and (5) a backbone of support organizations (Kania & Kramer, 2011). Collective impact initiatives also employ eight key principles that support population-level change: (1) designing and implementing initiatives with a focus on equity; (2) including community members; (3) cocreating initiatives with cross-sector partners; (4) using data to support continuous learning and improvement; (5) involving leaders with systems leadership skills; (6) focusing on program and system strategies; (7) growing relationships, trust, and respect among all partners; and (8) customizing initiatives to the local community (ORS Impact & Spark Policy Institute, 2018). These principles can guide social entrepreneurs and their collaborators in structuring partnerships for maximum impact.

### *Communities of Practice*

One way to strengthen the impact of collective impact initiatives is to build communities of practice where leaders and practitioners of change learn from and with each other as they work toward large-scale social change (Boyea-Robinson, 2016). Communities of practice are groups of people who share a common concern, problem, or passion about a topic and aim to increase their knowledge and expertise by interacting on an ongoing basis (Wenger et al., 2002). Communities of practice support the long-term, dynamic work involved in changing systems. Over time, communities of practice support the development and distribution of collective understanding and practices derived from both tacit and explicit knowledge (Meagher-Stewart et al., 2012). Sharing tacit knowledge requires interaction and informal learning (Wenger et al., 2002). Research has indicated that tacit knowledge can be preferred by practitioners and is critical to decision-making in initiatives in public health (Meagher-Stewart et al., 2012). Sharing practice-related stories, challenges, and circumstances leads to robust discussions around what efforts have already been applied and what strategies can be employed to influence change. The success of communities of practice hinges in part on the ability of participating partners to "fail forward" by sharing their struggles and failures along with their successes so that members can learn and advance the practice (Edmondson & Hecht, 2014). The community of practice framework can offer social entrepreneurs and their collaborators opportunities to expand their networks, share knowledge across systems, and identify innovative solutions to address social issues.

### *Authentic Leadership*

Leadership serves as a driving force to push innovative ideas forward and serves a pivotal role in the success and impact of social entrepreneurship. Leadership in social entrepreneurship is about helping others to envision a new possibility, "appreciate its meaning, and recognize how it can be broken down into doable steps that build momentum for change" (Bornstein & Davis, 2010, p. 25). Social entrepreneurs demonstrate persistence, resourcefulness, care, and attention to detail to see ideas through to completion. They must attract a following that will help the initiative to gain momentum through the participation, funding, and resourcing needed to get innovative ideas off the ground—while working through a range of responses toward the proposed change and attending to needs and issues as they arise to keep forward momentum.

Leaders in social entrepreneurship favor collaborative approaches and distributed leadership. They recognize their limitations and strengths and build complementary partnerships that help to advance social change. They are emotionally intelligent and strive to be genuine, authentic, and transparent in their approach to leadership. Authentic leadership offers a leadership framework that is centered on these qualities (George, 2015; George et al., 2007). Authentic leaders continually learn through actively embracing insight-oriented principles that focus on personal experiences, motivations, and values (George et al., 2007; George, 2015). In new situations, authentic leaders work to draw from their core values and principles and their past experiences, while also learning from new colleagues (George, 2015). Authentic leadership is about being true to oneself, building trusting relationships, and leading with integrity and purpose. It is an integrated approach to leadership that emphasizes the importance of self-awareness, ethical behavior, and genuine connection with others. Authentic leadership aligns with the ethical and transparent approach to leadership which is pivotal to success in social entrepreneurship and can help to guide leaders through the challenges and opportunities that arise in this work.

## ABOUT THIS BOOK

Modern-day trailblazers in the field of art therapy have narratives about their work and a drive toward change that energizes us. They inspire us to think about possibilities for our field and the communities we serve. Listening to art therapy colleagues talk about their innovative approaches, new programs, and initiatives has been something I look forward to at our professional conferences. Though I had created new programs and services in my career both as an intrapreneur and entrepreneur, I never associated with these terms. It was not until I was approached by a leader within an organization where I was working who suggested, based on what they knew about me and my work, that I might be interested in the present entrepreneurial opportunity. The lens of entrepreneurship was a new way for me to conceptualize my work. I was inspired to curate panel discussions presented at the American Art Therapy Association annual conferences in 2020 and 2021 to highlight innovation and social entrepreneurial practice in art therapy (DeLucia et al., 2020, 2021). Many of those panelists are contributing authors to this text. I hope that you find inspiration in the entrepreneurial activities shared by contributing authors, as I have, and that this inspiration contributes to an expansive view about what is possible when we utilize our skills as art therapists to tackle social issues in meaningful and sustained ways.

Art therapists frequently pioneer inventive approaches to tackling social problems that impact the communities they serve. They actively engage with issues of equity, inclusion, and accessibility by pioneering programs, grassroots advocacy, and policy initiatives. Chapter 1 situates art therapy within the field and practice of social entrepreneurship. In Chapters 2–11, the authors illustrate how their entrepreneurial endeavors in art therapy have generated significant social impact, contributing to the advancement of equitable and inclusive practices. The chapter authors describe how they identified the opportunity or need, the vision for their program or initiative, their implementation process, how they addressed risks, and discuss the skills and strategies they employed to promote success.

Chapters 2 and 3 are both notable examples of intrapreneurship and demonstrate that you do not need to start a new organization to be a social entrepreneur. These examples highlight how questioning the status quo, challenging assumptions, and learning about root causes and systems surrounding social challenges can illuminate opportunities to mobilize resources in new ways to address those challenges. These chapters provide examples of how this work is accomplished through partnerships, interdisciplinary collaborations, and building power for others.

In Chapter 2, Emily Goldstein Nolan describes Culture Circle Studios, a program designed to promote healthy relationships within a success center program operating in a public school by supporting behavioral change, mental health, and emotional literacy and regulation through restorative practices. The program provides a space for people working within the school to explore their assumptions about education and discipline practices. The goal of the program was to produce systemic and cultural change. As a result of the success of the initial pilot, the program was expanded district-wide. Nolan describes how her dual perspective and experience as an art therapist and former art educator helped her to identify the need she addressed and to propose a solution that would attend to the challenges, concerns, and potential limitations of the setting. She also provides examples of strategic partnerships and how she aligned with the mission and goals of the setting to achieve buy-in and participation. Action research was used to assess and respond to challenges and to drive change.

In Chapter 3, Mary Andrus presents the formation of Art for Social Change, an art activism group at a U.S. college. Andrus discusses issues of power within academia and provides the reader with an orientation to the social and cultural issues and events that served as the impetus for forming Art for Social Change. This chapter provides an example of how a two-year PAR project shaped the initiative to be more liberatory and anti-oppressive by creating spaces for collective healing, action, and trust. Interdisciplinary partnerships and engagement across the three campuses of the college brought together a diverse group of students, staff, faculty, alumni, and community members to participate in Art for Social Change. This chapter highlights how the initiative expanded and was sustained through an off-campus space, embedded in the community, where it incorporates a public practice art therapy model.

Chapters 4, 5, and 6 present examples of social entrepreneurial initiatives that address the needs of underserved and marginalized communities. In Chapter 4, Mitra Reyhani Ghadim and Rose Ehemann discuss the flourishing of the Living Museum. Reyhani Ghadim demonstrates how an established social entrepreneurial initiative of the early 1980s, the Living Museum, evolved and expanded to include contemporary art therapy approaches within its original structure, as well as expanding internationally to add Living Museums worldwide. Rose Ehemann, who is the founder of Living Museum in Wil, Switzerland, describes how starting the Living Museum in Wil led to the development of a nonprofit organization and a fundraising effort that supported the launch of five additional Living Museums in Switzerland. The authors discussed how they promoted and implemented new programming within existing institutions to expand the impact of the Living Museum model.

In Chapter 5, Chandra Davis describes an art therapy practice she founded on liberatory-based healing and intersectionality theory. She discusses how she infused these practices into her business in an intentional way, threading them through all her marketing materials, related advocacy and community outreach, and the services she offers. She shares marketing strategies and provides a case study that demonstrates how she integrates intersectionality and liberatory healing in her work with individuals in art therapy.

In Chapter 6, Lisa Lounsbury presents an overview of her experience developing a mobile art therapy facility to increase access to art therapy services in rural and underserved areas. She describes how she developed partnerships to support various phases of the project.

Chapters 7, 8, and 9 describe initiatives that target broader system-level concerns related to diverse representation in the field, as well as access to and standardization of art therapy services. These chapters highlight how the authors brought existing resources together in new and innovative ways to address macro-level needs within the field of art therapy.

In Chapter 7, Zachary D. Van Den Berg describes the formation of the Coalition for Queer Creative Arts Therapies (C-QCAT) and its annual digital event, Expressing Pride, highlighting them as examples of social entrepreneurship propelling queer creative arts therapies forward. They discuss how community participation and feedback were used to guide a community-oriented approach to moving the organization forward and address issues of sustainability.

Chapter 8 is coauthored by a group of art therapists who formed the Nebraska Art Therapy Licensure Coalition (NATCL) and coordinated advocacy efforts across Nebraska to successfully establish state licensure for art therapists practicing in the state. Their success story highlights an example of social entrepreneurial efforts focused on policy change to increase access and standardization of care for residents across a state. Their initiative serves as an excellent example of extrapreneurship, illustrating how resources can be pooled together across organizations to create an impactful systems-level change.

In Chapter 9, I frame the development of a new online graduate training program at an R1 research university as a form of social entrepreneurship targeting the need for accessible learning opportunities. A hybrid low-residency program was created to provide access to a wider range of students, reducing barriers to education that some students experience with attending a traditional on-campus program. Innovative and collaborative approaches to designing and implementing curriculum are discussed.

Chapters 10 and 11 provide examples of art therapy social enterprises. These are businesses operating with the primary goal of achieving social value while at the same time generating revenue.

In Chapter 10, Pamela Whitaker describes how Groundswell, an initiative in rural Ireland that is focused on environmental enhancement through the art of gardening, partnered with local and national government agencies to promote psychosocial support through art therapy and address the needs for rural development. She identifies how enterprise thinking guided the extension of Groundswell into public health, higher education, and climate action initiatives.

In Chapter 11, Emery Hurst Mikel provides inspiration and guidance to art therapists seeking to develop their own therapy practices as social entrepreneurs, taking us on a journey through the development of her two interrelated businesses. She candidly shares risks, doubts, and strategies that led to her success, discussing how her initiative to make art therapy more accessible for older adults in assisted living facilities led to the creation of her first business, Water & Stone PLLC.

In Conclusion, I conclude the book, by highlighting key points and suggestions for future directions for the field. I make a case for including social entrepreneurship in art therapy curriculum by weaving it with existing curriculum requirements focused on ethics and professional orientation to the field, as well practicum and internship experiences.

The first time when I heard the words "art" and "therapy" used together I had a light bulb moment that this field was my calling. Similarly, when I heard the term "entrepreneurial" in relation to my work it ignited a profound shift in how I perceive my role as an art therapist. Reflecting on the growth and evolution of the field over the years, I now see many of these efforts within the framework of social entrepreneurship. I hope that readers find the same level of inspiration in these concepts and case studies and envision how they might leverage social entrepreneurship to further the field and practice of art therapy.

## REFERENCES

Allen, P. B. (2011). Special issue on the social action and advocacy paradigm in art therapy: The lens of art therapy opens larger still. *Art Therapy: Journal of the American Art Therapy Association, 28*(2), 48–49. https://doi.org/10.1080/07421656.2011.579892

American Art Therapy Association. (2017). *About art therapy.* Retrieved September 30, 2024, from https://arttherapy.org/about-art-therapy

Armstrong, A. J., Holmes, C. M., & Henning, D. (2020). A changing world, again: How appreciative inquiry can guide our growth. *Social Sciences and Humanities Open, 2*(1), 100038.

Beugre, C. (2016). *Social entrepreneurship: Managing the creation of social value.* Routledge.

Bornstein, D., & Davis, S. (2010). *Social entrepreneurship: What everyone needs to know.* Oxford University Press.

Boyea-Robinson, T. (2016). *Getting back to the purpose of collective impact* [Blog Post]. Retrieved from https://collectiveimpactforum.org/blogs/28291/getting-back-purpose-collective-impact

Chahine, T. (2023). *Social entrepreneurship: Building impact step by step* (2nd ed.). Routledge.

Cooperrider, D. L., & Whitney, D. (2005). *Appreciative inquiry: A positive revolution in change.* Berrett-Koehler.

Dees, J. G. (2001). *The meaning of "social entrepreneurship".* Retrieved September 30, 2024, from The Meaning of Social Entrepreneurship | CASE (duke.edu)

Dees, J. G., & Anderson, B. B. (2006). Framing a theory of social entrepreneurship: Building on two schools of practice and thought. In R. Mosher-Williams (Ed.), *Research on social entrepreneurship: Understanding and contributing to an emerging field* (pp. 39–66). Aspen Institute.

DeLucia, J., Mikel, E., Lombardi, R., Nolan, E., Dejkameh, M., & Davis, C. (2020). *The act of creation: Art therapist as entrepreneur* [Panel presentation]. American Therapy Association 51st Annual Conference.

DeLucia, J., Royster, R., Lounsbury, L., Andrus, M., & Stallings, J. (2021). *Creative change agent: Therapist as entrepreneur* [Panel presentation]. American Therapy Association 51st Annual Conference.

Edmondson, J., & Hecht, B. (2014). Defining quality collective impact. *Stanford Social Innovation Review, 12*(4), 6–7. Retrieved from https://ssir.org/articles/entry/defining_quality_collective_impact

George, B. (2015). *What does authentic leadership really mean?* HuffPost: The Blog. Retrieved from www.huffingtonpost.com/bill-george/what-does-authentic-leade_b_8581814.html

George, B., Sims, P., McLean, A. N., & Mayer, D. (2007). Discovering your authentic leadership. *Harvard Business Review, 85*(2), 129–130, 132–138, 157.

Hanleybrown, F., Kania, J., & Kramer, M. (2012). *Channeling change: Making collective impact work* [Blog Post]. Retrieved from www.ssireview.org/blog/entry/channeling_change_making_collective_impact_work

Jackson, L. (2020). *Cultural humility in art therapy: Applications for practice, research, social justice, self-care, and pedagogy.* Jessica Kingsley.

Kania, J., & Kramer, M. (2011). Collective impact. *Stanford Social Innovation Review, 1*(9), 36–41.

Kapitan, L. (2018). *Introduction to art therapy research* (2nd ed.). Routledge.

Kaplan, F. (2007). *Art therapy and social action: Treating the world's wounds.* Jessica Kingsley.

Kummitha, R. K. R. (2017). Social entrepreneurship, community participation, and embeddedness. In R. K. R. Kummitha (Ed.), *Social entrepreneur and social inclusion* (pp. 33–52). Springer. https://doi.org/10.1007/978-981-10-1615-8_2

Lepoutre, J., Justo, R., Terjesen, S., & Bosma, N. (2013). Designing a global standardized methodology for measuring social entrepreneurship activity: The Global Entrepreneurship Monitor social entrepreneurship study. *Small Business Economics, 40*, 693–794.

Meagher-Stewart, D., Solberg, S. M., Warner, G., MacDonald, J., McPherson, C., & Seaman, P. (2012). Understanding the role of communities of practice in evidence-informed decision making in public health. *Qualitative Health Research, 22*(6), 723–739.

Merriam-Webster. (2023). *Merriam-Webster.com dictionary.* Retrieved September 30, 2024, from www.merriam-webster.com

Mohedano-Suanes, A., & Benitez, D. G. (2018). Intrapreneurs: Characteristics and behavior. In A. Tur Porcar & D. Ribeiro Soriano (Eds.), *Inside the mind of the entrepreneur: Cognition, personality traits, intentions, and gender behavior* (pp. 109–119). Springer.

Mulgan, G. (2006). The process of social innovation. *Innovations: Technology, Governance, Globalization, 1*(2), 145–162.

Nandan, M., Bent-Goodley, T. B., & Mandayam, G. (2019). *Social entrepreneurship, intrapreneurship, and social value creation: Relevance for contemporary social work practice.* Washington, DC: National Association of Social Workers.

Nicholls, A. (2006). Introduction. In A. Nicholls (Ed.), *Social entrepreneurship: New models of sustainable social change* (pp. 1–35). Oxford University.

ORS Impact & Spark Policy Institute. (2018). *When collective impact has an impact: A cross-site study of 25 collective impact initiatives.* Retrieved from http://orsimpact.

com/DirectoryAttachments/2262018_103655_540_CI_Study_Report_February_2018.pdf
Paul, T., & Neil, S. (2017). Social innovation: A window on alternative ways of organizing and innovating. *Organization & Management, 19*(1), 51–60.
Short, J. C., Moss, T. W., & Lumpkin, G. T. (2009). Research in social entrepreneurship: Past contributions and future opportunities. *Strategic Entrepreneurship Journal, 3*, 161–194.
Sparviero, S. (2019). The case for a socially oriented business model canvas: The social enterprise model canvas. *Journal of Social Entrepreneurship, 10*(2), 232–251.
Talwar, S. K. (2018). *Art therapy for social justice.* Routledge.
Tasker, M., Westberg, L., & Seymour, R. G. (2010). Action research in social entrepreneurship: A framework for involvement. *International Journal of Action Research, 6*(2–3), 223–255.
Thompson, J., Alvy, G., & Lees, A. (2000). Social entrepreneurship—a new look at the people and potential. *Management Decision, 38*(5), 328–338.
Wenger, E., McDermott, R. A., & Snyder, W. (2002). *Cultivating communities of practice: A guide to managing knowledge.* Boston, MA: Harvard Business School.
Zahra, S. A., Gedajlovic, E., Neubaum, D. O., & Sculman, J. M. (2009). A typology of social entrepreneurs: Motives, search processes and ethical challenges. *Journal of Business Venturing, 24*, 519–532.

*Chapter* **1**

# Creative Changemaker

## Art Therapist as Social Entrepreneur

*Jennifer Marie DeLucia*

### ART THERAPISTS AS SOCIAL ENTREPRENEURS

In a post-pandemic era, we understand more than ever that the future is unpredictable and that we need to have the ability to be adaptable and flexible. Art therapists develop and hone these qualities through the experience of being practicing artists. For example, most artists are familiar with working with ambiguity and imperfection while remaining open to emerging possibilities. Rarely do artistic creations materialize in the exact way we imagined, without some struggle with execution. One reason is that artistic vision often exceeds artistic skill. When making art, art therapists work through stuck points and respond repeatedly to unexpected results, developing a tolerance for the unknown through this process. Art therapists often transform "mistakes" or "failures" in art into expressive and impactful imagery and objects, in their own art and when working with people in communities and therapeutic settings. It is the nature of the art therapist to promote experimentation with materials and to make room for failure, helping people to view failure as an opportunity rather than a setback.

The training and education of artists cultivates a unique perspective and way of seeing. Artists develop observation skills through intentional examination of details such as shape, form, and color. For example, an artist may see the edges of an object and interpret the shape in a more accurate way than a person without this formal training. Art therapists are trained to hone their assessment skills through observation, active listening, empathy, and cultural competence. The ability to observe and perceive issues beyond what is visible at the surface is a key skill in social entrepreneurship. Creativity and an ability to envision new possibilities are equally

DOI: 10.4324/9781032615776-2

important. Successful innovators simultaneously perceive ground-level views of problems and a blue-sky vision. They can bring people together and encourage experimentation and creativity.

A social entrepreneur's goal is that the new ways of addressing social problems they develop take root and change behavior and thinking (Bornstein & Davis, 2010). This is no small task. System changers must overcome "apathy, habit, incomprehension, and disbelief while facing heated resistance from those with vested interests" (Bornstein & Davis, 2010, p. 22). Creativity, resourcefulness, and innovation are key elements of entrepreneurship that are most relevant to social entrepreneurs (Nicholls & Cho, 2006). These characteristics parallel many of the traits held by art therapists, who are trained to be creative, resourceful, and innovative in their work with individuals and communities. Art therapists have a deep understanding of the process of change management and of the persistence and creativity needed to sustain the motivation to change. Art making is an essential component of how they promote development in the people and communities they serve (Kaimal et al., 2017). Art therapists use art making and the creative process to help people envision possibilities for the future, to see problems from multiple perspectives, and to identify incremental steps toward change. Using parallel skills, social entrepreneurs are "change agents for society, seizing opportunities others miss and improving systems, inventing new approaches and creating sustainable solutions to change society for the better" (Nicholls & Cho, 2006, p. 102).

Effective leaders and system changers possess an embodied knowledge that has less to do with intellectual knowledge than it has to do with personal attributes such as decisiveness, compassion, enthusiasm, persuasiveness, and the ability to listen, to be firm, to establish boundaries for others, and to inspire (Ibbotson, 2008). Social entrepreneurs are persistent in their approach and remain open to adapting their ideas as needed to address concerns and needs of the system they are working within. Social entrepreneurs initiate and guide transformative processes that are inherently adaptive, geared toward growth, and centered on making a meaningful impact. These processes involve forming new collaborations among individuals and orchestrating collective efforts to address challenges (Bornstein & Davis, 2010). The social entrepreneur, like the art therapist, helps others to envision a new possibility, understand the meaning and potential impact of doing things in a new way, breaks change down into small achievable steps, and celebrates small successes to build momentum for change.

New ideas that achieve social impact have a reliable and persistent driving force that provides "care, energy, resourcefulness, and stubbornness necessary to navigate the idea through the system" (Bornstein & Davis,

2010, p. 23). Social entrepreneurs must attract attention and funding, shift behavior, and mobilize political will, continually improve the idea, and meticulously take care of all details, no matter how long it takes (Bornstein & Davis, 2010). Entrepreneurs tend to have a strong inner locus of control. They believe that if they do not have the skills or resources to solve a problem, they can acquire them through learning, experimenting, observing experts, and seeking help (Bornstein & Davis, 2010). They view failure as something that can be addressed with more specialized knowledge and effort. Similarly, art therapists often promote a greater sense of internal locus of control through the therapy process. They emphasize clients' agency and self-efficacy, holding an optimistic perspective that change is possible. They are flexible in their approach to working with individuals and communities, understanding the balance needed to motivate people toward the goals they seek to achieve. Art therapists are skilled at applying consistent effort over a long period to promote change.

It has been said that artists may experience failure more than any other group. Bouncing back from perceived failures and moving forward with creativity and persistence are at the heart of the creative process. Artists are accustomed to taking risks. They take risks in creating by trying new techniques, styles, or mediums and by pushing the boundaries of their art. They take personal and emotional risks by sharing their thoughts, feelings, and perspectives through their artwork, potentially making them vulnerable to rejection and criticism. Social entrepreneurs assume similar risks and, like artists, must persevere through discomfort and potential rejection to see ideas through to completion, reframing perceived failure as an expected part of the process and using knowledge gained to iterate on solutions and move ideas forward. Art therapists exhibit many of the traits central to success in social entrepreneurship, and viewing their work through this lens can highlight new potential for leveraging the resources needed for social impact.

## ART THERAPISTS' BUSINESS, LEADERSHIP, AND ENTREPRENEURIAL SKILLS

In 2024, I distributed a survey designed to explore art therapists' experiences with leadership, business, and entrepreneurship. The survey examined seven related skills and nine personal characteristics related to business, leadership, and social entrepreneurship that were commonly found in the literature (DeLucia & Linsner, 2025).

Seven skills were identified in the literature associated with social entrepreneurship, and the survey was constructed to ask the same five questions about each skill. The seven skills included: (1) resource management, (2) vision and goal-setting, (3) key partner and community engagement, (4) creating innovative solutions, (5) measuring outcomes, (6) resource mobilization, and (7) strategic communication. Each skill was briefly defined in the survey. Participants were asked if they had experience using that skill, what type of related training they may have received, how their experience as an artist contributed to their development of that skill, how their experience as a therapist contributed to the development of that skill, and how often they use that skill in their current position.

The second section of the survey had participants use a five-point scale to rate how much they demonstrate the following characteristics: (1) persistent, (2) adaptable, (3) resilient, (4) good listener, (5) skilled negotiator, (6) organized, (7) comfortable with uncertainty, (8) able to deal with setbacks, and (9) capable of finding joy in small successes. Participants were then asked how much their experience as an artist has supported the development of these traits, and how much their experience as a therapist has supported the development of these traits.

The perspectives shared revealed how participating art therapists viewed their work, practice, and training as artists and therapists as providing them with experience related to these skills and characteristics. Some of the skills resonated more with participants' experiences as artists or therapists than others, though all skills prompted some level of reflection on the potential areas of overlap. The following provides an overview of the qualitative data collected in the open-ended questions regarding each of the seven skills identified in the literature.

## Resource Management

In social entrepreneurship, resource management involves efficient and effective planning, allocation, and utilization of various resources to align with and achieve set goals (Yoganandan & Dinesh Kumar, 2023). Resources can include but are not limited to human resources (e.g., people), financial resources (e.g., funding), physical resources (e.g., facilities), material resources (e.g., supplies), partnerships (e.g., collaborations), nonmonetary contributions (e.g., volunteer efforts), and time. Several art therapists who participated in the survey felt that their experience as artists contributed to the development of creative problem-solving skills and "out-of-the-box thinking" required for resource management. They described how identifying materials for making art in resource-constrained environments, utilizing materials in inventive ways to compensate for limited financial resources, and budgeting for costs of materials were specific ways their experience as practicing artists supported their development of skills related to resource management. Similarly, social entrepreneurs are skilled at assessing available resources and bringing them together in new combinations and ways to achieve their socially oriented goals.

Social entrepreneurs, like artist therapists, often operate in resource-constrained environments and rely on their own personal credibility and professional networks to garner support for new initiatives with a socially oriented mission (Swanson & Zhang, 2012). Art therapists identified their interpersonal effectiveness skills, such as conflict management and active listening, as key supports in their development of skills in resource management. They also described how their work as therapists cultivated a high level of patience and an optimistic disposition that supports them in managing limited resources, being resourceful, and advocating for art therapy. A primary task of art therapists is to establish trusting relationships with the people they work with to enable self-expression (Kaimal et al., 2017). Skills identified by art therapists align with those needed to cultivate support for new ideas and solutions in social entrepreneurship. Social entrepreneurs must "capture the imagination of a community of supporters through the combination of contagious courage and pragmatic persistence" (Mulgan, 2006, p. 153). They must also establish a sense of trust and confidence among key partners and communities of interest.

### Vision and Goal-Setting

Vision and goal-setting involve envisioning a new possibility, understanding the impact of doing things in a new way, breaking change down into small achievable steps, and celebrating small successes to build momentum for change (Bornstein & Davis, 2010). As artists, art therapists have developed skills for identifying an artistic vision and mapping steps to achieve that vision. These skills were acquired within their individual art practices and are used when working with groups and communities. Art therapists also identified that art making itself facilitated vision and goal-setting by using art making as a way of clarifying intentions, goals, and aspirations.

Art therapists lead change processes that are growth-oriented and seek to achieve a desired outcome or impact. Many art therapists who responded to the survey identified skills in treatment planning and goal-setting with clients as directly related to the development of this skill. They also identified how they used various therapeutic approaches such as positive psychology, motivational interviewing, cognitive behavioral therapy, and client-centered approaches to support vision and goal-setting with others. Personal development through consultation with other professionals and interpersonal effectiveness skills were also identified as supporting the development of vision and goal-setting skills.

Emotional intelligence—which includes self-awareness, self-management, social awareness, and the ability to manage relationships—supports success in social entrepreneurship (Xie et al., 2018). Like the art therapist, the social entrepreneur must thoughtfully navigate change and maintain positive relationships with key partners, employing effective interpersonal skills and maintaining a high level of self-awareness. Art therapists are well positioned to leverage their skills and experiences as therapists to inform and enhance their vision and goal-setting processes in various personal and professional contexts. Art therapy education prepares art therapists to "understand human experiences within sociopolitical and cultural contexts" promoting empathy and understanding of diverse experiences (Kaimal et al., 2017). Through a client-centered approach, utilization of therapeutic techniques, integration of positive psychology, and commitment to continual learning, art therapists strive to achieve their aspirations and facilitate growth in themselves and others.

## Key Partner Engagement

A key partner is anyone who will influence or is influenced by the outcome, decisions, or activities associated with a project or intervention. Key partners can be funders, volunteers, community members, the intended beneficiaries of the intervention, or people who are engaged in implementing the solution. Key partner engagement involves understanding community needs, preferences, and ideas for solutions, and is accomplished by bringing people together to exchange knowledge about the identified problem. This engagement is important because key partners contribute resources to support the success of the social entrepreneurial initiative. As such, all key partners' needs and perspectives have to be considered when making decisions and working to achieve outcomes (Smith & Woods, 2015).

Art therapists who participated in the survey described how attunement to the needs of others and society more broadly is a function of being an artist. As artists, they routinely consider the perspectives of those receiving, purchasing, or exhibiting their artwork, as well as the intended audience. As therapists, they identified several interpersonal effectiveness skills they have mastered (such as active listening, asking open-ended questions, and seeing things from multiple perspectives) that supported key partner engagement. Several art therapists noted that they routinely engage with multiple key partners as therapists, considering the needs, strengths, values, and motivations of the client, the setting where the services are delivered, and the broader community. When I think about my own practice as an art therapist, I reflect on working with youth and families. When the needs and interests of the youth are not aligned with the goals of the parent(s), the therapist must attend to both perspectives to keep everyone invested in continuing therapy. The ability to psychologically hold and attend to different (and at times competing) interests is a skill central to key partner engagement in social entrepreneurship.

### Creating Innovative Solutions

Creating innovative solutions involves developing new, original, and effective approaches to addressing challenges or meeting identified needs. Developing innovative solutions requires thinking outside the box, being adaptable and open to feedback, and integrating feedback through problem solving, experimentation, and refinement. Innovation is at the heart of social entrepreneurship, and is likewise at the center of artistic practice. There were many survey responses from art therapists who stated that being an artist *is* being an innovator. Artists often engage in an intuitive process of trial and error, experimenting and refining as they develop their craft. They engage in creative problem-solving as identified by survey participants who noted their skill and ability as artists to think expansively, approach problems with curiosity, and improvise. Participants identified that artists are accustomed to taking risks and developing their willingness to try different approaches without being discouraged. In social entrepreneurship, creating innovative solutions is an iterative process, and it does require a level of comfort with risk-taking; planning for a process that involves failure, feedback, and improvement.

Therapeutic skills and training were identified by participants as supporting innovation. This included an ability to tolerate ambiguity, being able to hold multiple viewpoints at once, using positive psychology techniques to enhance positive emotions and expand creative thinking, and working with clients to find new ways to overcome barriers. Like skilled therapists, successful social entrepreneurs are "good at talking and listening, digging below the surface to understand peoples' needs and dislocations, dissatisfactions, and blockages" (Mulgan, 2006, p. 150).

### Measuring Outcomes

Measuring outcomes refers to evaluating the results, impact, or effects of an intervention, program, or project. It involves establishing clear objectives and developing methods to collect and analyze information regarding how well the objectives are being achieved. Art therapists most identified with how their training and experience with developing goals for therapy and treatment plans relate to this skill, as well as their backgrounds and training in program evaluation. Experiences with developing measurable outcomes in art therapy training and practice directly translate to measuring outcomes in social entrepreneurship, particularly when paired with art therapists' ability to assess needs at multiple levels within a system. Art therapists also identified that their interpersonal effectiveness skills and their ability to view change and progress in multiple ways contribute to this skill area. Viewing progress in multiple ways also relates to skills and training as an artist. Participants identified that creativity and the ability to think outside of the box help with developing outcome measures that are not constrained by dichotomous thinking. Using visual tools in the distribution of outcome data is a skill related to their training or practice as artists and their ability to identify ways to visually represent information in an impactful way.

### Resource Mobilization

Resource mobilization refers to acquiring new resources or leveraging existing resources in a new way that helps the organization, program, or project achieve its goals. Unlike resource management, discussed earlier, which focuses on the utilization of existing resources, resource mobilization focuses on securing additional resources required to support an initiative. As the terms are closely related, some of the responses art therapists provided regarding resource management overlapped with responses to resource mobilization. However, some distinct contributions were noted. Art therapists identified that in their work as therapists they were regularly required to think creatively to identify resources. Limited resources made it necessary for them to seek alternative solutions and advocate on behalf of the individuals and communities served for increased support. Interpersonal effectiveness skills include empathy, compromise, negotiation, active listening, and communication skills used to develop relationships. These skills, as well as case management skills, were described as helpful in mobilizing resources. One participant identified that they learned about grants and funding opportunities on the job to help mobilize additional financial resources to support programming.

### Strategic Communication

Strategic communication refers to deliberate and planned communication conveying information that aligns with the goals of the organization, program, or project. It involves tailoring messaging to meet the needs and interests of different key partners and communities of interest and leveraging communication strategies to advocate for increased support or promote awareness. Strategic communication skills resonate with the experiences of many participating art therapists, who observed that their skills in observation, interviewing, and developing therapeutic working relationships were highly related. Art therapists highlighted the importance of understanding and using various forms of communication, including nonverbal cues and tailored approaches to effectively interact with clients, treatment teams, and other key partners in therapeutic settings. Effective communication skills were identified as essential for conveying messages accurately, advocating for clients' needs, and navigating complex systems such as insurance and institutional policies. There were also parallels to their art-making practices, as one art therapist identified that "engaging in the creative process with a clear intention and care is to practice strategic communication."

## FRAMING SOCIAL ENTREPRENEURSHIP IN ART THERAPY

Social entrepreneurship requires a balance between business priorities and social priorities (Alter, 2006; Neal, 2015). Many art therapists serving in leadership, management, and administrative roles are required to use business skills such as financial management (budgeting, reporting), general management (building and maintaining relationships with key partners, allocating and overseeing the use of financial and human resources), leadership (motivating and mobilizing people toward a common goal), strategic planning (developing and achieving goals for 3–5-year plans), and negotiation. Even when not serving in a formal leadership capacity, art therapists benefit from having skills to navigate the political and business aspects of working in organizations. Art therapists are often pulled into making decisions related to funding and marketing in various settings and find themselves navigating the space between ethical art therapy practice and the business practices and priorities that support sustainability.

Mainstream conversations about social entrepreneurship have emerged from the fields of business, public health, and public policy, and business schools offer the primary opportunities for curriculum and professional development in social entrepreneurship (Neal, 2015). Business jargon may not resonate with many people working in the helping professions (Neal, 2015). However, it is complicated to fully untangle business issues and art therapy practice when art therapists are increasingly involved in seeking funding and reimbursement for services, developing new programs within existing organizations, and advocating for policy change. Social entrepreneurship offers a framework that brings together the social interests of people working in helping professions with business practices that can be leveraged to effect change.

Art therapists may not view themselves as social entrepreneurs. However, many are well suited to the relational and creative abilities required for this role. Art therapists can assess the needs of their community and develop ways to innovate programming and services in meaningful and systemically impactful ways. Establishing new ways of practicing, building programs to address unmet needs, and contributing to the growth of the field through job creation all support increased access to art therapy services. Participatory approaches to assessing needs and working *within* communities can increase access and address issues related to equity in mental healthcare. Further, deliberate approaches across mental health settings can promote institutional change, adaptation, and innovation, addressing gaps in service delivery (Exton, 2008). Adapting how art therapy services are offered demands integrating creativity with entrepreneurial skills and finding ways to draw from both established and innovative practices.

Art therapists are driven by both a personal calling and ethical responsibility to enhance the welfare of others. The *Ethical Principles for Art Therapists*, published by the American Art Therapy Association (2013), has established principles that guide art therapists' decision-making with core values that support ethical practice. The preamble lists seven core values that include autonomy, nonmaleficence, beneficence, fidelity, justice, and creativity. The guiding value of beneficence is described as the ways that art therapists "promote wellbeing by helping individuals, families, groups and communities to improve their circumstances" and "enhance welfare by identifying practices that actively benefit others" (p. 1). The value of justice describes how art therapists "commit to treating all persons with fairness" and "ensure that clients have equal access to services" (American Art Therapy Association, 2013, p. 1). The ethical principles described include a responsibility to the profession centered on art therapists participating in activities that advance the goals of art therapy. As stated, "art therapists value participation in activities that contribute to a better community and society" and "recognize the importance of developing laws and regulations pertaining to the field of art therapy that serve public interest, and with changing such laws and regulations that are not in the public interest" (American Art Therapy Association, 2013, p. 11).

Literature in the field of social work identifies how social entrepreneurship aligns with social work's values of service, social justice, and competence (Nandan et al., 2019; Neal, 2015; Pitt-Catsouphes & Berzin, 2015). Like social work, the field of art therapy is rich with examples of social entrepreneurship, though not conceptualized through this framework. Viewing these examples through the lens of social entrepreneurship can expand opportunities for specialized training and mentorship to support these initiatives. Neal (2015) identified the power of social entrepreneurship to augment social work practice, empower clients, provide alternative funding sources, and offer insulation from disruption of essential services. Arguably, this is true for the field of art therapy as well.

Bent-Goodley (2002) defined social work entrepreneurship as "the creation of institutions through entrepreneurial thinking that are guided by social work ethics and based on the integration of social service, business, and public relation skills" (p. 291). They also discussed the barriers to entrepreneurship in social work, including a perception that being business-focused is incompatible with maintaining professional social work ethics. One aspect of this is related to concerns that social work should focus on altruism and not financial gain. There are ethical considerations in operating a business; however, an individual can be highly ethical and entrepreneurial at the same time, if the needs of the communities served are properly addressed. A final barrier Bent-Goodley addressed was the need to balance social work curricula to address the needs of students, the profession, people served, and society. They challenged the notion that students should be trained to work only within established institutions and added that opportunities can be introduced to train students to create and sustain entrepreneurial ventures.

Curriculum requirements in art therapy leave little space to add new content in required courses. However, programs may consider adding elective courses that cover related content. When programs do not have the resources to develop new courses alone, they might partner with other programs on campus. Given the alignment of social entrepreneurship with our ethical standards and the realities of the practice landscape, there will be a continued need and opportunity for new professionals to lead in entrepreneurial ways. Though not all students may be interested in or well-suited to serve the field as entrepreneurial leaders, training opportunities will provide them the opportunity to understand the foundational elements and skills required to be successful. The field of art therapy and communities served by it will also benefit as new generations of art therapists enter the field prepared to navigate entrepreneurial opportunities.

The frontline perspective of many art therapists provides them with a vantage point and understanding of unmet needs and opportunities that may be more insightful than the top-down or outsider perspective of many funders and community development corporations. As the field of art therapy continues to grow and evolve, the competencies required to practice must follow. I predict that with an increased focus on community-based art therapy, the skills associated with social entrepreneurship will be increasingly seen as valuable foundational skills that need to be introduced in graduate training programs.

## REFERENCES


Alter, S. K. (2006). Social enterprise models and their mission and money relationships. In A. Nicholls (Ed.), *Social entrepreneurship: New models of sustainable social change* (pp. 205–232). Oxford University Press.

American Art Therapy Association. (2013). *The ethical principles for art therapists.* Retrieved from https://arttherapy.org/wp-content/uploads/2017/06/Ethical-Principles-for-Art-Therapists.pdf

Bent-Goodley, T. B. (2002). Defining and conceptualizing social work entrepreneurship. *Journal of Social Work Education, 38,* 291–302.

Bornstein, D., & Davis, S. (2010). *Social entrepreneurship: What everyone needs to know.* Oxford University Press.

DeLucia, J. M., & Linsner, R. K. (2025). Creating impactful change: An exploration of art therapists' experiences related to social entrepreneurship. *Art Therapy: Journal of the American Art Therapy Association,* 1–13.

Exton, R. (2008). The entrepreneur: A new brand of health service leader? *Journal of Health Organization and Management, 22*(3), 208–222.

Ibbotson, P. (2008). *The illusion of leadership.* Palgrave Macmillan.

Kaimal, G., Metzl, E., & Millrod, E. (2017). Facilitative leadership: A framework for the creative arts therapies. *Art Therapy: Journal of the American Art Therapy Association, 34*(3), 146–151.

Mulgan, G. (2006). The process of social innovation. *Innovations: Technology, Governance, Governance, 1*(2), 145–162.

Nandan, M., Bent-Goodley, T. B., & Mandayam, G. (2019). *Social entrepreneurship, intrapreneurship, and social value creation: Relevance for contemporary social work practice.* National Association of Social Workers.

Neal, A. A. (2015). The intersection of social work and social enterprise. *Journal of Social Work Values & Ethics, 12*(2), 1–9. Retrieved from www.jswve.org/wp-content/uploads/2015/12/10-012-201-JSWVE-2015.pdf

Nicholls, A., & Cho, A. H. (2006). Social entrepreneurship: The structuration of a field. In A. Nicholls (Ed.), *Social entrepreneurship: New models of sustainable social change* (pp. 99–119). Oxford University Press.

Pitt-Catsouphes, M., & Berzin, S. C. (2015). Teaching note—incorporating social innovation context into macro social work education. *Journal of Social Work Education, 51,* 407–416.

Smith, L., & Woods, C. (2015). Stakeholder engagement in the social entrepreneurship process: Identity, governance, and legitimacy. *Journal of Social Entrepreneurship, 6*(2), 186–217.

Swanson, L. A., & Zhang, D. D. (2012). Social entrepreneurship. In T. Burger-Helmchen (Ed.), *Entrepreneurship: Gender, geographies, and social context* (pp. 171–190). InTech.

Xie, X., Lv, J., & Xu, Y. (2018). The role of the entrepreneurial personality in new ventures. In A. T. Porcar & D. R. Soriano (Eds.), *Inside the mind of the entrepreneur: Cognition, personality traits, intention, and gender behavior* (pp. 99–108). Springer.

Yoganandan, G., & Dinesh Kumar, M. (2023). Qualities of successful entrepreneurs—a review of relevant literature. *Materials Today: Proceedings, 81,* 173–175.

Chapter 2

# Culture Circle Studios

## Unifying a School Community in Healthy Relationships[1]

*Emily Goldstein Nolan*

### INTRODUCTION

I have been a student and an educator my whole life. I am also a parent of children in the educational system. Before I became an art therapist and art therapy educator, I was an art teacher in both public and private schools. I know that as a young teacher, I did not understand the importance of teaching through a relational model, which is a model that centers the child and how the child perceives and relates to important adults as allies and advocates. My professional growth, curiosity, drive to feel competent, and failed interactions with tough students (those who challenged the rules and were constantly needing redirection) led me to seek better ways of classroom management. A supportive school social worker helped me see the importance of creating positive connections with students; this was my responsibility as the teacher and adult. I sought out information about how to create positive relationships with students. As I practiced using the knowledge, classroom management became easier, and students met academic and classroom goals.

As my relationships with students grew and deepened, I felt the focus of my work shifting to their emotional experiences within the school system and in their home and community environments. I saw that those experiences were affecting their academic performance and their overall health. As a teacher, even with better skills in place to develop positive relationships with students, I felt I could be even more effective if I became an art therapist and art therapy educator. Although I could not see this almost 25 years ago, these were formative experiences that influenced me in creating the Culture Circle Studios, or CCS.

DOI: 10.4324/9781032615776-3

The CCS are designed to provide a space for school administrators, educators, and staff members to explore their assumptions and experiences about education and discipline practices with the intention to bring about systemic and cultural change in their workplace environments. The CCS were designed initially to promote an atmosphere centered around healthy relationships in the Success Center (SC) program at Green Bay Avenue School in the Milwaukee Public School District (MPS) in partnership with Marquette University Center for Peacemaking, Bloom Art and Integrated Therapies, Inc., and several other therapeutic partners. The CCS program was implemented with the intention of innovating an application of art therapy services to a new practice area, providing professional development, and training in using action research to carefully develop new programming.

## SUCCESS CENTER MODEL

The SC program is a therapeutic school program that offers art therapy, yoga, dance/movement, and drumming as well as traditional mental health therapy to students and their families. The program targets 3rd through 12th grade students who are underfunctioning in the academic setting and who may have some underlying behavioral and mental health concerns. Students leave their school of origin to participate in the program for a period of nine weeks. Using a restorative model, which uses many tools to create an overall culture of care, the goal of SC is to interrupt the school-to-prison cycle which affects a disproportionate number of marginalized youth (Garnett et al., 2019; McCluskey et al., 2008; Sellman et al., 2013; Wadha, 2016). The culture created within the SC program is empathetic and the restorative model is enacted through a focus on creating careful healthy relationships to prevent conflict and behavioral concerns. Many processes and interventions, called circles, are used to repair harm, help the student be successful, and transition back to their school of origin.

The faculty and staff of the SC program are working through challenges of innovating a new model of education that addresses mental health and supports behavioral change, emotional literacy, and regulation through restorative practices. The restorative model of education begins with the faculty and staff creating intentional and supportive working relationships with each other and modeling that for the students and their families. As they create this culture of support within the program as a whole and with families, they are challenged with seeding this cultural shift back at the home school of the child so that growth gains are maintained. The program overall seeks not only to impact students and families but also to influence the larger school system, supporting teachers and all schools in MPS beyond the SC.

During the COVID-19 pandemic, as the founder of Bloom Art and Integrated Therapies, and developer of the art therapy program for the students at the SC, I had the opportunity to sit in on many of the faculty and staff virtual meetings at the SC. During that time, I noticed that the educators were all passionate about their work with students but were lacking in relational skills. The SC brought educators together, but as a group they seemed disjointed and lacked a sense of cohesion. They not only did not work effectively as a team, but some of the educators did not know how to approach a dysregulated student without becoming highly dysregulated themselves or understanding that their assumptions about students influenced how they interacted with them. While my BFA in art education had not included training in creating healthy relationships, I had received training in healthy relationship skills during graduate school, and I have taught the Helping Relationship and Applications in Art Therapy class for two different graduate art therapy programs since 2011. I began to think intentionally about the needs of the SC and my skills. I wanted to provide an opportunity for the SC educators to develop their relational skills and support the goals of this new program. I thought about how to address the need for community within the SC and how to support the educators in centering students through engaging in healthy relational interactions with them and each other. In attending many of the SC meetings, I had built positive relationships with many of the faculty, staff, and administrators within the center and the MPS district. I proposed the Culture Circle Studio, first to the SC administrators and partner, Marquette University Center for Peacemaking. In addition to being the founder of Bloom, I am a faculty member at Syracuse University. I wrote a faculty enrichment grant to fund an initial pilot program to implement Culture Circles at the SC, which was funded by the College of Visual and Performing Arts. The grant allowed me to make personal art kits for each participant in the study and funded the additional art supplies for the circles.

Once I developed the art therapy program for the SC, the administrators asked if they could apply the therapeutic structure of that program to the overall SC model. The administrators started to consult with me more often on the SC's creation and refinement. They began to understand the need of the adult community of the SC and the skills that I had to share. The administrators at the SC and this author invited faculty and staff to participate in the CCS.

Each adult at the SC went through the CCS to promote an inclusive relational culture of accepting one another and relating to each other in healthy ways. The SC endeavors to provide a different approach to working with one another, the students and families, and the system to encourage a thriving educational climate and culture. My work centers on building healthy relationships to foster acceptance, inclusion, and belonging, and advocates for change. It is through relationships that any change toward growth can be leveraged. The SC aspires to center healthy relationships with students and families while students are brought through a process that helps them to reorient their response to classroom learning and to regulate their nervous systems. The behavioral changes and regulation students experience enhance their ability to attain success in the classroom setting and school environment. However, once the student returns to their school of origin, their overall success is dependent on the other people and environments in the educational system changing with them. Herein lies a challenge: to support the sense of community among the SC adults and students, and then spread that to the schools of origin and district schools.

In general, schools and school districts are a part of a larger system of interacting values and dynamics. A school has its own values and expectations and is made up of a community of people embedded in a larger community and society. Maintaining awareness of how a school and the school system are placed within the larger system while facilitating the circle process can provide important context. Understanding what participants in the circle may be bringing with them as experiences or underlying assumptions is helpful, as these contribute to the culture of the school. Here, culture is viewed as "a multidimensional phenomenon that encompasses processes, products and results of human activity, material and spiritual" (Mironenko & Sorokin, 2018, p. 338) passed on from generation to generation. According to Fullan (2007), school culture can be defined as the guiding beliefs and values evident in the way a school operates. School culture encompasses all the attitudes, expected behaviors, and values that impact how the school operates. The culture circles seek to change school and district culture over time, through centering health relationships.

The CCS process supports and examines the adults' experiences, including staff, teachers, and administrators in the educational setting, and offers skills to build and maintain beneficial relationships that encourage optimal conditions for learning. The goal of the CCS is to promote healthy cultural and systemic change in the schools and throughout the district that centers relationships to achieve student success. This chapter outlines the development of the CCS program from one that was offered to the faculty and staff at the SC, then expanded to other educators in the district, and finally, to being employed as a task-sharing model that trains educators in the district to facilitate the culture circles. My strategic implementation and development of the program sought to widen the circle of cultural change.

## EMERGENT DATA AND ACTION RESEARCH

The Office of Research Integrity and Protections and the Institutional Review Board at Syracuse University reviewed and approved the CCS protocol. Action research was used to develop the CCS program and to gain systemic change through the implementation of each set of circles themselves (see Figure 2.1). Action research was initially developed by Kurt Lewin (1946) as a research model to "emphasize making an immediate difference in the world" (Willis & Edwards, 2014, p. 11). Action research is a systematic form of investigation and "typically involves attempts to solve practical problems in real world settings through the involvement of stakeholders who work or live in those settings" (p. 19). Action research takes place within practice settings. The purpose of action research is to change how practice is conducted, the understanding of practice, and/or the environments where the practice happens (Kapitan, 2018). Action research methods promote reflexive practitioners who embrace reflection in action and who adopt a research mindset in observing and acting upon their

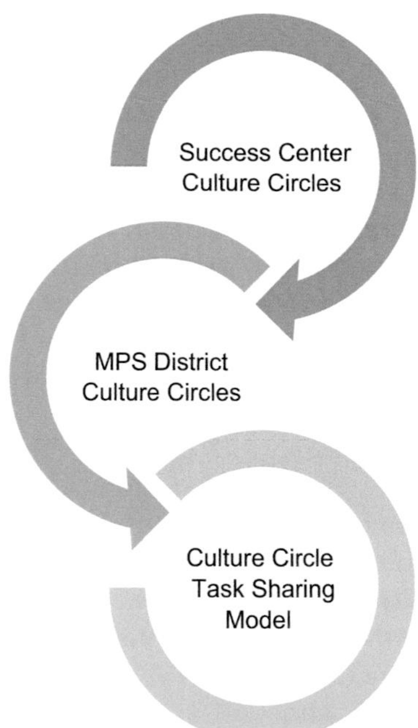


***Figure 2.1*** *Culture Circle Studios (CCS): Action Research Cycle Progression.*

*Note*: Action research was used to develop the CCS program and to gain systemic change through the implementation of each set of circles.

environments to create affectual change. Action research can be used in art therapy program development to assess needs, implement interventions based on those needs, observe the effects of the intervention, evaluate the effectiveness, and refine the program offering (Nolan, 2023).

Critical cultural circles are a type of action research with a specific structure that includes a collective cycle of reflection, naming, dialogue, and action (Magill & Rodriguez, 2019; Friere & Macedo, 2005). Culture circles are used in education and are based on Friere's concept of conscientization, or awareness raising, which leads to social change (Souto-Manning, 2010). Culture circle facilitators are there to help groups gain awareness of their potential and capacity for transformational action. Facilitators use arts-based research (ABR) to support group members as they work through questions designed to raise their awareness of their actions, increase their ability to attend to healthy relationships, and develop their commitment to change. ABR uses art processes within a research framework (Barone & Eisner, 2012; Kapitan, 2018; Leavy, 2020), and is based on the understanding that "art is both an object and event that invites . . . transformation, . . . healing and reconciliation" (Kapitan, 2018, p. 218).

When implementing ABR, art making can be used for data gathering, data analysis, and in presenting and disseminating findings of the research (Kapitan, 2018).

Art-based inquiry in the culture circles generated ideas, deepened meaning, and identified actions to create change in the educational environments at the SC and throughout MPS.

In each of the sessions of the Circle, participants use art as a form of inquiry. The participants work together on a large wooden panel with a circle drawn upon it; they follow prompts to stimulate visual thinking and place their images on the panel. After the session, the facilitator visually responds to the images on a separate panel (see Figure 2.2). The first session introduces the participants to the circle process and the use of art as a form of research and as a method for visual thinking. The first session sets up the visual framework of knowing, meaning-making, and understanding for the subsequent sessions. The second session seeks to generate themes from the participants' experiences of education and their taken-for-granted educational and discipline/punishment practices. The third session identifies problems within the school system through deconstructing the participants' narratives on how the social structure of education has influenced participants' realities, why they think school-based punishment and discipline happen the way they do, how those practices affect the classroom and school dynamics, and how these practices affect the overall program and district culture. The fourth session is for dialoguing and considering the multiple perspectives of each participant and collectively constructing knowledge about education that is relevant to each

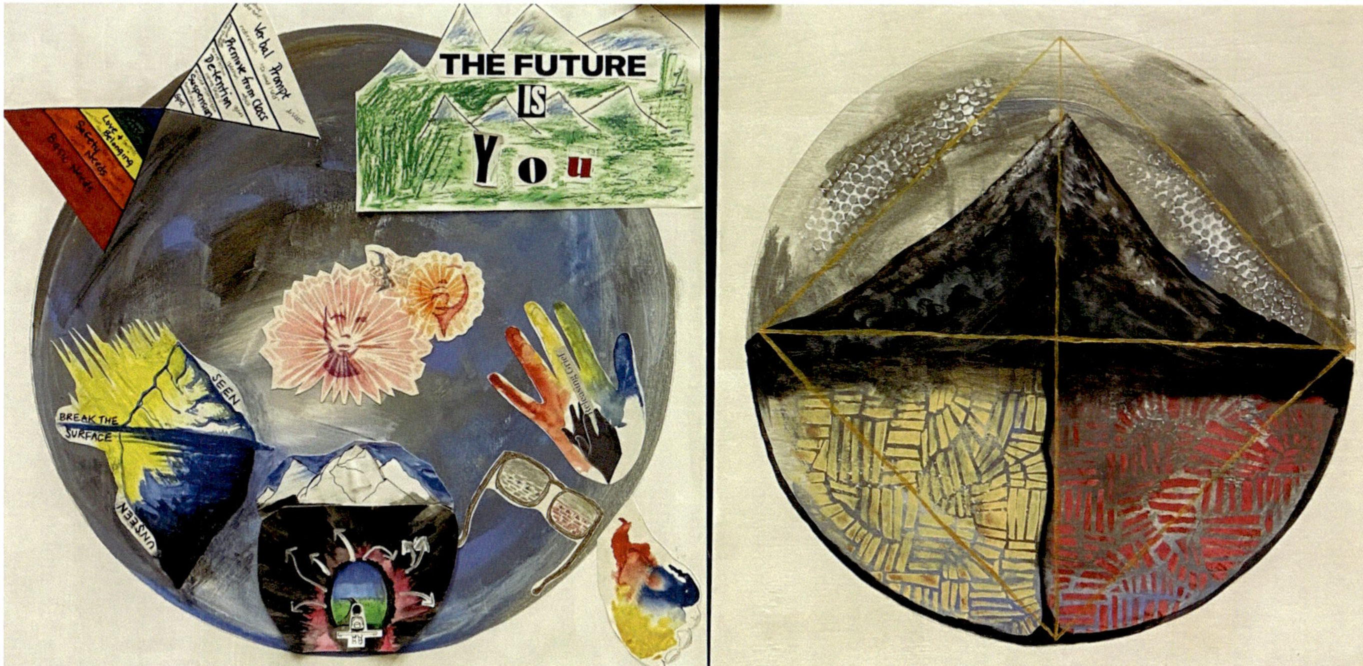


*Figure 2.2 Call and Response.*

*Note.* Panel A (left) shows the art-based inquiry results of the participants' images and symbols used to represent their experiences in education. Panel B (right) illustrates the facilitator's response as the synthesis and amplification of those images and the reflexive dialogue with participants.

person's experience and reality. The fifth session is for problem solving, collectively dreaming about what can be done to create change. The sixth session focuses on the actions each person is willing to take to effect change. All remaining sessions are committed to supporting the educators' actions for change, very much like how art therapists participate in arts-based supervision as a new professional.

## CULTURE CIRCLES

### Round 1: Culture Circles Within the SC

The culture circles were first implemented at the SC in the spring of 2021. The circles were supported in part by the Marquette University Center for Peacemaking and a faculty enrichment grant through the College of Visual and Performing Arts at Syracuse University, and were conducted through Bloom Art and Integrated Therapies, Inc. Two cohorts of faculty, administrators, and staff from the SC program completed the circle process. One cohort was led by this author and the other cohort was led by Erica Browne. Erica is the lead art therapist in the SC program and the Executive Director of Bloom. Erica attended the first cohort as a participant, and then worked with this author to facilitate the sessions for the second cohort. The MPS schools were just beginning to return to in-person sessions in the spring of 2021, following COVID-19 restrictions, and the sessions took place once per week for 7 weeks.

### Round 2: Culture Circles for the School District

After feedback from the participants of the initial SC culture circles, and with the encouragement of the MPS administration, Bloom was invited to provide the CCS to other teachers, staff, and administrators across the school district. District administrators invited any staff, teacher, or administrator from the SC student participants' schools of origin to participate in the CCS. This call to the schools of origin yielded enough participants to fill two cohorts. Participants included paraprofessionals, teachers, trauma specialists, discipline specialists, and school social workers. Art therapist Amber Thomas, an employee of Bloom, used the CCS curriculum to lead the two cohorts through the culture circle process. The cohorts used the prompts from the first program to creatively process their experiences in education, encourage change, and support one another. The cohorts met once per week for 7 weeks and were invited to attend additional support sessions. One of the trauma specialists who attended this round of the CCS asked to meet with me about other options for bringing adults in the district through the culture circle process. That conversation resulted in the district inviting me to create a task-sharing model for the circles. The task-sharing model would offer a train-the-trainer process, bringing district support staff (such as trauma and discipline specialists) through a training where they could facilitate the circle process at the schools where they were associated. The train-the-trainer process would offer more access to the circles and, in effect, increase the pace of district change.

### Round 3: Culture Circle Studios Tasking Sharing Model

This third, task-sharing, round of CCS was made possible through the Elementary and Secondary School Emergency Relief Fund (ESSER) Funding provided to MPS. The U.S. Department of Education provided ESSER funding to schools for support during the COVID-19 pandemic, and CCS programming was funded under ESSER as professional development. Prior to offering the task-sharing model, I wrote a manual and curriculum for the training and self-published using Kindle Direct Publishing to cost-effectively provide materials for the cohort and offer the information to other school districts.

A task-sharing model is a structured way to educate professionals to provide services when a more well-qualified or skilled professional is unavailable (Keshri & Garg, 2021; Orkin et al., 2021). Art therapists are uniquely positioned as facilitators for the CCS program because of their professional use of the creative process in art-based inquiry, their knowledge of group facilitation, and their skills in developing healthy relationships. MPS has few art therapists available to provide CCS, and this training is an opportunity to shift culture and contribute to a healthy community within the school district by employing adjacent professionals in the role of facilitator, without needing to be an art therapist. It is important to note that support professionals who participated in this training were clearly informed that they are not able to function in any capacity as an art therapist after program completion. After the program, they can lead CCS within MPS. Participants in the training explored the elements and skills of facilitating a CCS for others, experienced the process themselves, and were supported while facilitating CCS in their areas. The first ten sessions led facilitators-in-training through experiencing a CCS, while also exploring the skills and concepts they would need when facilitating their own sessions. In the final ten sessions, professionals processed their own experiences leading the circles and asked for feedback when needed.

## Art Prompts and Materials

This section covers the art prompts I developed for use in CCS session, as well as the art materials that should be provided to each participant. While I was developing the art prompts, I thought about the concepts I wanted us to examine and how to creatively use the critical cultural circle process. I considered not only my own experiences as an educator and art therapist, but what I had observed and learned from staff, educators, and administrators over the years.

### *Session Art Prompts*

1. Create an image of your best self in the schools.
2. Create an image that contemplates your experiences of discipline in education as a child and an adult.
3. Create an image of the problems you see in education related to punishment and discipline.
4. Create an image that explores the perspectives of all the people who make up the school environment.
5. Create an image that collectively dreams of how education could be.
6. Create an image of yourself as a superhero in education, what superpowers do you have?
7. Create an image of being relationally oriented.
8. Support Sessions: Create art related to maintaining healthy relationships, or anything else that you would like to process visually related to your setting.

### *Materials*

Each participant is given a personal art kit for use in and outside of the CCS. Additional supplies are provided by the facilitators to use during the circles to support artistic exploration.

#### The Art Kit

- 5 × 7 journal with mixed-media weight paper
- Pencil set
- Watercolor paint set
- Watercolor brushes

- Color pencils
- Markers
- Sharpies

**Additional Materials**

- Various types of paper (drawing, tissue, construction)
- Magazines
- Collage materials
- Stencils
- Scissors
- Precision knife
- Cutting board
- Glue
- Acrylic paints
- Acrylic brushes
- Oil pastels
- Rulers
- Water containers
- Paper towels

## DISCUSSION

I used many entrepreneurial attributes in developing the Culture Circle Studios. First, my efforts to mobilize change required that I gathered a team of like-minded people with similar goals. When Bloom Art and Integrated Therapies, Inc., was invited to develop the art therapy program for the SC, we realized there was a need for the schools to invest in professional development in building relationship skills among school professionals. The SC was founded on being relationally centered, which made it easy for us to assemble a team. As a team member, it was important for me to listen to the needs key partners brought forth during each cycle. Key participants included MPS administrators, teachers, paraprofessionals, staff members, social workers, psychologists, trauma specialists, discipline specialists, and therapists as well as representatives from Marquette University and SC administrators. Centering these relationships meant the circles attended to needs they identified, which included the need for more support resources, especially in the realm of community care and self-care.

After implementing each round, I carefully observed how the circles were received and valued by the participants. I paid attention to how the changes from the circle affected others in the district, either through their observations of change or their interactions with the participants of the circles. I adjusted each round and further refined the circles to meet the emergent needs. For example, one of the administrators of the SC was initially reticent to participate in the CCS. Once he began attending, he really engaged in the process and saw the impact the circle had on helping him to identify the purpose of his work. He named his own experiences as a student and saw how those impacted his desire to help students be successful. After he went through the CCS, he became one of the biggest proponents for bringing the process to other educators in the district. With each round, we scaled up the program; the program started in the Success Center, moved beyond the SC to the district, and was then offered as a task-sharing model with a self-published facilitator's manual available for purchase on Amazon. The scaling-up effectively brings this model from impacting only one school program, to touching a whole district, and potentially reaching more schools and districts, widening the reach of systemic change.

## CHALLENGES

The biggest overall challenge of the project has been one of change. Change takes time, and in a large, dynamic system, it can happen very slowly. Part of that change was asking teachers to buy into yet another professional development experience. Many times, professional development is a requirement placed on educators already being asked to do more with less. There are a record number of open positions at MPS, and new teachers seeking employment at MPS are at an all-time low. New teachers are also more likely to take a position at a more resourced and/or smaller district than MPS. MPS teachers often have large classroom numbers due to the shortage. Paraprofessionals are often used to fill staff shortages. Paraprofessionals do not need a teaching degree, which means undereducated individuals are filling in the gaps, doing more with less education. Also, many required professional development trainings are one-time experiences that deliver a set of expectations for teachers with no follow-up to support implementation. Inviting educators to one more training and getting them to buy in is difficult. Their reticence to participate is understandable given how much the school system has typically asked from them, and not provided needed support.

## CONCLUSION

By using a task-sharing model and action research to develop this program, we generated a multiplier effect and provided greater access to needed skills and support than we could have otherwise provided (Kapitan, 2006). When using a task-sharing model, it is important to consider how the information imparted during the training could be thinned out or watered down when implemented by non-art therapy professionals. The lack of experience with art therapy concepts, combined with the skills the non-art therapy professionals bring, could ultimately weaken the experience of the group members who participate in future circles.

I believe there is a set of skills and knowledge that art therapists can offer in non-treatment settings, such as those developing as art therapy grows as a field and art therapists innovate programming outside of medical settings and in the community. Art therapists are trained to create healthy relationships, think visually, and use art to determine problems and goals. Action research provides a logical framework for developing new art therapy programming. Using action research to develop and evaluate programs is systematic, yet naturally fits with building new programs. Art therapists can try out new ideas and then critically reflect on what is observed as a result.

Using an action research mindset ethically considers sustainability in that art therapists draw from the resources of the community where the program is implemented. Art therapists are often in situations where they are invited to create new programs with limited resources. Using action research, the art therapist can carefully consider what resources are available to draw upon in the community and use those in planning and action cycles.

In this chapter, I reflected on my efforts to implement a professional development experience that helps the adults working in public schools to build healthy relationship skills using art-based inquiry and to create intentional feelings of belonging in the community. I used action research with entrepreneurial concepts to create programs to accomplish these goals. I gathered a team to mobilize efforts and create effective change, and then scaled the program appropriately to provide skills to the designated professionals. Art therapy is growing as a field and, as it does, there are myriad ways it can be functionally applied to new arenas. When art therapy is used innovatively and implemented strategically, art therapists extend the reach of the field and the benefits to more people.

## NOTE

1 Some of the information in this chapter can also be found in the self-published manual I wrote for training others to lead Culture Circle Studios. Nolan, E. G. (2023). *Culture circle studios: Unifying a community of supportive administrators, educators, and staff in healthy relationships*. Kindle Direct Publishing.

## REFERENCES


Barone, T., & Eisner, E. (2012). *Arts-based research.* Sage.

Friere, P., & Macedo, D. (2005). *Literacy: Reading the word and the world.* Routledge.

Fullan, M. (2007). *The new meaning of educational change.* Routledge.

Garnett, B., Smith, L., Kervick, C., Ballysingh, T., Moore, M., & Gonell, E. (2019). The emancipatory potential of transformative mixed methods designs: Informing youth participatory action research and restorative practices within a district-wide school transformation project. *International Journal of Research & Method in Education, 42*(3), 305–316. https://doi.org/10.1080/1743727X.2019.1598355

Kapitan, L. (2006). The "multiplier effect": Art therapy research that benefits all. *Art Therapy, 23*(4), 154–155. https://doi.org/10.1080/07421656.2006.10129336

Kapitan, L. (2018). *Introduction to art therapy research* (2nd ed.). Routledge.

Keshri, V., & Garg, B. (2021). Operational barriers in providing comprehensive emergency obstetric care by task shifting of medical officers in selected states of India. *Indian Journal of Community Medicine, 6*(2), 252–257. https://doi.org/10.4103/ijcm.IJCM_563_20

Leavy, P. (2020). *Method meets art* (3rd ed.). The Guilford Press.

Lewin, K. (1946). Action research and minority problems. *Journal of Social Issues, 2*(4), 34–46.

Magill, K., & Rodriguez, A. (2019). Culture circles as a practice of freedom. *Curriculum and Teaching Dialogue, 21*(1/2), 53–70.

McCluskey, G., Lloyd, G., Stead, J., Kane, J., Riddell, S., & Weedon, E. (2008). "I was dead restorative today": From restorative justice to restorative approaches in school. *Cambridge Journal of Education, 38*(2), 199–216. https://doi.org/10.1080/03057640802063262

Mironenko, I., & Sorokin, P. (2018). Seeking for the definition of "culture": Current concerns and their implications: A comment on Gustav Jahoda's article "critical reflections on some recent definitions of 'culture'". *Integrative Psychological Behavior, 52,* 331–340. https://doi.org/10.1007/s12124-018-9425-y

Nolan, E. G. (2023). *Community art therapy: Theory and practice.* Routledge.

Orkin, A., Rao, S., Venugopal, J., Kithulegoda, N., Wegier, P., Ritchie, S., VanderBurgh, D., Martiniuk, A., Salamanca-Buentello, F., & Upshur, R. (2021). Conceptual framework for task shifting and task sharing: An international Delphi study. *Human Resources for Health, 19*(61), 1–8. https://doi.org/10.1186/s12960-021-00605-z

Sellman, E., Cremin, H., & McCluskey, G. (Eds.). (2013). *Restorative approaches to conflict in schools: Interdisciplinary perspectives on whole school approaches to managing relationships.* Routledge.

Souto-Manning, M. (2010). *Friere, teaching and learning: Culture circles across contexts.* Peter Lang.

Wadha, A. (2016). *Restorative justice in urban schools: Disrupting the school-to-prison pipeline.* Routledge.

Willis, J., & Edwards, C. (Eds.). (2014). *Action research: Models, methods, and examples.* Information Age Publishing.

Chapter 3

# Art Activism for Social Change

*Mary Andrus*

## ART ACTIVISM WITHIN ACADEMIA

In the United States, there are many art therapy master's and bachelor's degree programs that promote social justice in their marketing materials. Given the divisions within our country and ongoing societal rifts, as program director, I recognized the need for our program to engage in effective action toward activism. Specifically, steps toward creating equity, access, and building a community of future art therapists seeking the promotion of social justice. Thus, Art for Social Change was formed through the intention of creating a shared space to process and respond to ruptures in society, to build community, and use the art for healing. Art for Social Change is an art activism group that formed in 2020 on an American college campus. Our group is a collective of faculty, students, staff, alumni, and community members from diverse social backgrounds and demographic identities, encompassing biracial, multiracial, White, queer, Indigenous, and gender nonconforming individuals.

## ACADEMIA AND POWER

The United States is built on what Wilkerson (2020) defines as a caste system and has established social norms that privilege Whiteness. People are motivated to maintain their space and place in society by asserting power over one another through social, cultural, symbolic, and economic capital (Bonanno, 2018). Higher education in the United States is a system built on capitalism (Bullard, 2007) and has its roots in colonization (McMillan-Cottom, 2017). This capitalistic structure contributes to

DOI: 10.4324/9781032615776-4

hierarchical social capital (Şerban, 2023). Attending a higher education institution provides social prestige, in the form of institutionalized cultural capital through credentials, qualifications, and embodied capital in the form of skills (Kon, 2017). It also creates collective identity through shared cultural capital and space to build social capital through the relationships formed through the institution (Bourdieu, 1977). One's proximity to these expressions of capital translates into power, rank, and status. These societal messages are imprinted in the mind's eye of the normalizing gaze that categorizes people into groups in a socially created panopticon (White & Epston, 1990). These positions of power hold people in society and are dependent on a range of privilege reliant on others to keep their status (Stepney, 2022).

The field of art therapy is majority White and majority women (Awais, 2022). As a White, cisgender, nondisabled, middle-class, female art therapy program director, I acknowledge the importance of reflecting deeply on my own privileged relationship to power and motivations to do this work. I must engage in ethical practices that work to expand the field to include more diverse people who shift this demographic (Awais & Yali, 2013).

The field also has an ethical responsibility to move toward a decolonized version of therapy that embraces community-based practices and recenters the lived experiences of people who have historically lived in our society at the margins with a lack of power due to inherent racism, systemic discrimination, oppression, and injustice. To approach community-based practices ethically, we need to consider "regularly challenging biases through intentional, creative interaction with people who are dissimilar" to each other (Timm-Bottos, 2016, p. 161).

The art therapy field continues to pursue recognition as a legitimate, distinct discipline, working to gain respect and credibility in related fields, and not be viewed simply as a technique or intervention. This has resulted in pedagogy, accreditation requirements, and board certification standards that are directed toward an insurance-driven medical model or the "clinicification" (Allen, 1992) and less on process-focused approaches, i.e., somatic or community-based work. Art therapists are beginning to embrace a decolonized version of therapy (Kanerahtenhá:wi Whyte & Toll, 2023; Mandler McKnight, 2023). Editors of publications in the field are considering ways to move out of the modern lens into a post-structural epistemology that interrogates power, shifts away from focus on the individual, and works toward collective healing (Andrus, 2023).

Art therapy pedagogy that shifts away from rote memorization and focuses on in-depth education that explores power, oppression, and inequities within institutions can be transformative. Black feminist scholar bell hooks (1991) posits that there is no gap between theory and practice, that theory as a social practice can be liberatory. By engaging critical thinking instead of rote memorization, students can "connect what they learn to what it might mean to hold power accountable, address social injustices, and both imagine and struggle for a more just world" (McLean, 2015, p. 307).

Many Black art therapists have been doing community-based work for social equity, e.g., Cliff Joseph (1989), Georgette Seabrooke-Powell (Boston & Short, 2011), Lucille Venture (1977), and Sarah McGhee (Doby-Copeland, 2019), all whom have focused their careers in working with people in communities and advocating for social change. Unfortunately, their work and voices have been silenced and left out of art therapy graduate training.

There are many examples of how our society has failed its people and created structures that harm communities of people who are on or at the margins (Anzaldúa, 1987). The United States has multiple interconnecting structures based in capitalism (Sanders, 2023), and a known history of racism, sexism, discrimination, and violent genocide that are perpetuated within these structures. More recently, we have witnessed an increase in hate crimes (U.S. Department of Justice, 2024) and anti-trans legislation around the country (Trans Legislation Tracker, n.d.); and since the loss of Ruth Bader Ginsberg in 2020, there has been a majority conservative Supreme Court, resulting in increasingly restricted civil rights following their 2023 decisions, i.e., overturning *Roe v. Wade* (Totenberg & McCammon, 2022) and the end of affirmative action (Howe, 2023). Given what is happening in our society environmentally, politically, and interpersonally, we need social spaces to gather, mourn, process, reflect, share, witness, and heal.

Through the raised critical consciousness that emerged in the United States after the social and racial awakening in 2020, there has been a noticeable shift within publications that center anti-oppressive practices (Gopalakrishna, 2022; Van Den Berg & Allen, 2022; Wright & Wright, 2022). Art for Social Change was formed in an academic setting at Lewis & Clark College in Portland Oregon and emerged with the intent of creating an anti-oppressive structure. Next, I will share a bit about this place to give context to our story.

## PORTLAND

Portland is progressive and liberal; the people are passionate, creative, and embrace unique self-expression. In Portland, being queer or trans is welcomed and normed, people are caring, and naming pronouns is a common way of identifying oneself. The city has a dark history of colonization, land acquisition, supremacist formation of the Ku-Klux-Klan in the 1920s, and Black exclusionary laws that were created to specifically keep people of color out of Oregon (Camhi, 2020). It is a place where an armed group of far-right extremists took over the Malheur National Wildlife Refuge (Zaitz, 2016) and where extremist groups (like the Proud Boys) have engaged in violent gatherings and assaults on demonstrators (Flaccus, 2019).

I have witnessed people of color fighting for their right to be treated equally, unjust targeting by Federal law enforcement (Wilson, 2022), and a city of progressive passionate activists who were the center of media attention during the pandemic (Killen, n.d.). This resulted in Portland being viewed as a dangerous place, where Antifa, riots, and looting still permeate people's minds (Brooks, 2023). In 2020, there was intense media attention on Portland, where protesters marched for 100 days straight. Peacefully protesting people were pulled into unmarked vans and arrested by plain-clothed officers (Levinson et al., 2020). Police used tactics such as tear gas and rubber bullets that caused harm not only to protesters but also to residents in their homes (Dowling, 2020). Passionate activists included the "Wall of Moms," locked arms with matching yellow t-shirts, middle-class middle-aged white women activists, protesting police brutality (Kurtzleben, 2020), accompanied by the DADBlock known for wielding leaf blowers in response to the tear gas (Lang, 2020). Even after four years, a negative public perception of Portland still lingers (Brooks, 2023).

Post-pandemic, like other major metropolitan cities in the United States, Portland's inhabitants suffered from a loss of jobs and the lack of affordable housing (Hayden, 2023). What emerged is very little separation of people with and without means, inhabiting the same geographic areas. Oregon ranks close to last in the United States when it comes to access to mental health (Ranking the states of 2022, n.d.) and last in regards to drug treatment services (Caballero, 2023). There is a significant need for care and a lack of resources, resulting in a large number of unhoused people living in recreational vehicles, on the streets, or in tents in unclaimed areas in neighborhoods around the city.

## LEWIS & CLARK

Lewis & Clark is an institution of higher education, located across three campuses in Portland, with roots and structure that emerged from colonization. It is dependent on tuition and private and government funding, often taking advantage of the labor of adjunct faculty to maintain its configuration. The institution was originally called Albany Collegiate Institute and was relocated to Portland in 1938; it was renamed in 1942 to Lewis & Clark (LC). There are many entanglements to navigate within what a name means to people. For some, it represents money, brand recognition, tradition, and a felt connection to a place; for others, it represents pain and harm.

The values of the graduate school are social justice, equity, and access. Under the leadership of LC's new president, Dr. Robin Holmes-Sullivan, the administration has been building scaffolding for holding difficult conversations within the institution. The administration has launched a series of listening sessions exploring the mascot, which is a Pioneer, or "Pio" for short. The term pioneer describes a settler or someone who migrated West to settle new territory. I believe these discussions are a safe way to begin exploring the dissonance of identifying as a forward-facing social-justice institution, with a name that, for some, represents a connection to colonization. I do believe they are working toward these ascribed values of social justice and equity; however, institutional change takes time and requires cycles of deep listening, understanding, and collective action.

## ART FOR SOCIAL CHANGE BEGINNINGS

The summer of 2020, after learning of George Floyd's murder, I had an intense somatic response resulting in creating a large piece of art (see Figure 3.1). Reflecting on the current social and racial unrest, and my privilege, responsibility, and social power as a program director, I believed it was important to move into action, mobilize, and bring people together, using art as a catalyst for change.

My identity as an art therapist is anchored in the act of creating art within a community and collaborating on art projects that engage people in collective action. During the time I was creating this artwork, Olivia 'Liv' Siulagi (an art therapy alumni), her father Lawrence Siulagi (an employee at LC), and I formed Art for Social Change, with Lawrence and I serving as co-chairs.

Through discussions with students, we brainstormed forming this group to be responsive to injustice, using art as a catalyst for change. We invited people across the institution to join our work. The group consisted of a variety of people, including students, staff, faculty, alumni, and community members. We formed a website, wrote a mission statement, and began meeting weekly on video.

I recently interviewed Lawrence to include his voice in this chapter and asked him about why he joined Art for Social Change.

## INTERVIEW WITH LAWRENCE SIULAGI

*What follows is a transcription of my interview with Lawrence Siulagi (held November 23, 2023, via Zoom):*

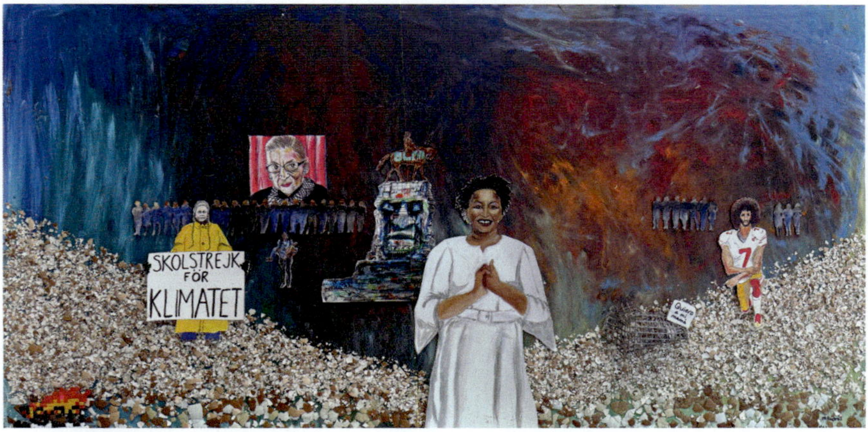


***Figure 3.1*** *"2020 in Hindsight" by Mary Andrus.*

*Note*: Mixed media on wood panel. A dark swirling oil paint forms the background and eggshells cover the ground, with the numbers 2020 on fire in the bottom left corner. Key illustrations, from left to right, depict Greta Thunberg in a bright yellow raincoat holding a sign that reads "Skokstrejk for klimatet;" a line of people marching; an image of Ruth Bader Ginsberg; a projection of George Floyd on the Robert E Lee statue; Stacy Abrams stands in the center foreground wearing a white dress clasping her hands together; a small cage with a sign that reads "Quiero a mi mama?;" and Colin Kaepernick kneeling in his uniform.

My name is Lawrence Siulagi, pronounced *See-eu-lung-ee.* I'm a communication specialist for the Office of Communications. I mainly work on the website. I am adept the Internet, and help manage information for the college brochure website. I'm part of a large office of communications team who, get along very well. And diversity is happening within little by little, which is very nice.

The reason why I got into Art for Social Change? The murder of George Floyd really sparked something in me, and I didn't have an outlet for that anger and the injustice of it. That's when I got the call from Olivia, from Liv, my daughter, who was learning [art therapy] in the grad school. And said, she was forming this group, along with you. [She said] "We really want to do something about it, and there's something we can do." So that's how it all started, bringing me into the group, and then I found that avenue of healing. That's what really attracted to me was the art part of it, because I'm a theater artist.

I'm Filipino, half Filipino, half Samoan, and my mother's Filipina, my Dad was Samoan. When they immigrated to the U.S. they really . . . they were not forced, but they chose to adapt to the dominant culture raising my sister and I, very White . . . in a very White environment in order to survive, or in order, maybe an admiration of proximity to whiteness. That was like a big thing for them, to at least for my mother. We didn't know our own language, I didn't speak Tagalog. I didn't speak Samoan. We weren't exposed to any type of teachings or even culture identity. I had really no identity at all except for confusion. [It resulted in me] really not knowing where I belonged. So, and because I was mixed race, even within people of color, it was even more difficult. We moved to Brazil for 4 years, and didn't even fit. I fit in otherwise, but I didn't fit in culture-wise, so that kind of became my culture. I've adapted in so many situations being a navy brat and stuff.

We lived in a racist society, but I wouldn't even call it that . . . I went to school, which was a very diverse school. When I lived in Brazil, of course it was very diverse, but most of the people there were White going to this American school, which was very expensive. I had great teachers and learned a lot. And then when I got back to San Diego, there's a lot of Latino and Black and Brown [people there]. It really wasn't until I moved to Portland, where it's like, yeah, this is, I feel definitely like, I'm a minority.

I felt that with art has no race, right? Art is just art, and it's an expression of higher power or expression, of spirit or expression of God or universe. And that is like the ultimate thing for me. For me. It's storytelling theater. I thought an Art for Social Change Group could be a place where I hear stories. I can also see stories and hear stories like through voice box, through drumming, through whatever, and that, you know the spiritual expression is infinite, so I can look at any type of art form. As a place to heal whether it's personal or whether it's global or universal, you know. So that's what attracted me to, because that was just a like a great fit. It's like, Wow! What a great thing, you know, Art for Social Change.

## LIBERATION PSYCHOLOGY

Initially, our group proposed to do large-scale projections or painted murals on campus that read "Black Lives Matter," "Silence Is Violence," and "Art For Justice." These proposed ideas were met with criticism from Black faculty and students, noting that engaging in these was performative allyship versus real change. They saw it as an empty gesture lacking institutional accountability. This feedback launched us into shifting our work and really taking a deep look at our motivations and what it means to engage in Art for Social Change.

Our group looked to liberation psychology to guide our work. The term liberation psychology was introduced by Martín-Baró (1994), who critiqued the epistemology of Western psychology, challenging positivism, individualism, hedonism, homeostatic vision, and ahistoricism. People who are oppressed engage in praxis, where they reflect and take action to change their world, transitioning from comprehension to transformation (Freiré, 2018). This reflection involves identifying their own conscious awareness of being in an oppressed group and the conscious awareness of the oppressor. This transforms into praxis when the group of oppressed people reflect collectively, engage in solidarity, and take action to fight against the oppressor. "The method lies in dialogue. They must fight for their liberation as the result of their own conscientização" (Freiré, 2018, p. 67). This critical consciousness-raising involves gathering in community to reflexively examine oneself in context, with dialogue and action. It is within this space, in praxis, where impactful change can occur.

Members in Art for Social Change began a two-year participatory action research project (PAR) that went through cycles of reflection, dialogue, and action, to shift our work to be more liberatory and anti-oppressive, engaging in building spaces for collective healing, collective action, and mutual trust (Andrus at al., 2024). We worked with psychodrama therapist and author Neito et al. (2010), curated a meaningful set of creative interventions to explore our motivations and how we navigate our work.

In our interview, Lawrence referenced a story told by Dr. Nieto that examined the ethos in the Pacific Northwest where peoples' interactions with each other created environmental conditions of it being "cold but nice," with an undercurrent of racism, and people of color not feeling welcome. He stated:

> And yeah, [I] remember that story. And just feeling like my nervous system was just . . . I couldn't even put it. I just didn't know. You don't know what you don't know. And it's kind of walking around, not feeling like completely deregulated. Because I can code switch. I can, you know, adapt.
>
> But there was always this feeling of just . . . it's very peripheral, psychologically peripheral vision of being feeling a little bit unsafe and then convincing myself that I could be safe. So when it came to George Floyd, everything just sprang up.
>
> And you know, I'm a person of color that's just been my life right? It should adapt. And really look at racism as like, okay, well, it's a problem. But I still have to work within a system that's already in power. Right? There's nothing I can do to control that. But I can do what I can through art and healing. And the ultimate protest is through art. I think you know, that is ultimately the thing.

## ACTIVISM OR PERFORMATIVE ACTIVISM?

Art has the potential to be utilized as "a radical pedagogical practice and strategy" (McLean, 2015, p. 311). Our shared vision was to bring together the three Lewis & Clark campuses and unify us through art, engage with the Portland community, and support work by people of color who were engaging in art as a catalyst for change. It was through our PAR study exploring the work of Art for Social Change where we used the process to inform our growth and the evolution of our organization.

After getting the feedback about the potential harm and performative activism of painting text on campus, we thought deeply about our work.

Personally, this feedback opened my eyes to my inclination as a White-bodied person to move toward action to feel good about myself rather than considering the harm or the perspective of others.

We created spaces for community building, healing, and reflection during our weekly open studio and established an annual Winter Solstice cleansing event. We created ties beyond campus with the larger Portland community, and supported a Black Portland activist who organized several Black Lives Matter art therapy events in community parks and donated supplies. We promoted events on social media and offered free materials and space to people who had been protesting. We hosted sewing circles, inviting community members to create a pandemic quilt (Figure 3.2), which reflected on the inequities and injustices within society—especially for BIPoC communities—that were revealed by the pandemic. We spent a year developing our land acknowledgments, working with Indigenous community members.

We actively discussed being at a college that promotes social justice and the optics of being dependent on and embedded in an institution named after colonizers. The dilemma of the name Lewis & Clark is bigger than the institution itself. We are aware that unless we are Indigenous people or are a descendant of people who came here against their will,

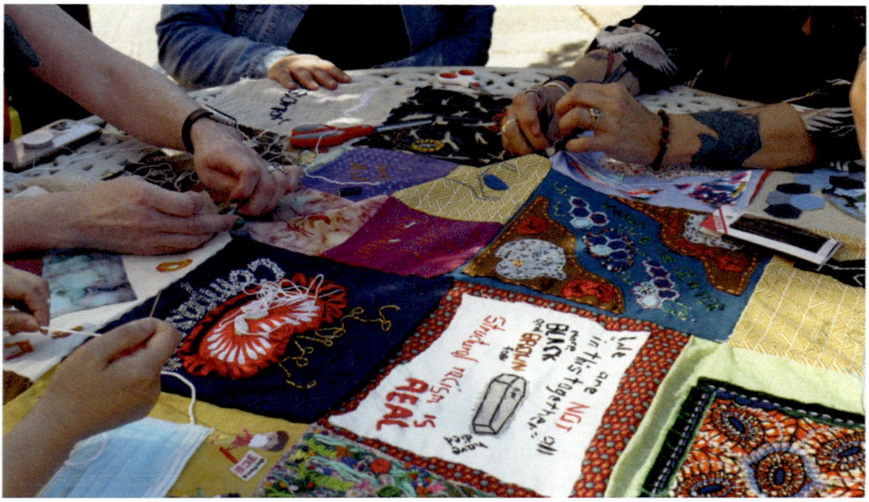


***Figure 3.2*** *Pandemic Quilt.*

*Note*: A photograph of ASC members working on a quilt on a table with four people working on stitching the squares together. Quilt squares range in color and design with the words "Love, Compassion" and "We are not all in this together, more black and brown folk have died. Structural racism is REAL." Photograph taken by Lawrence Siulagi.

we are still living on stolen land, still actively colonizing. We have learned to take a step back and restate our mantra to "move at the speed of trust" (brown, 2017).

Over time, as we evolved, we developed a structure for organizing our meetings. Based on the outcomes from our PAR study, we incorporated a structure that allows for shared leadership, shared responsibility, and shared input. We started every meeting reading our land acknowledgments, group agreements, and our mission statement, so as to remain rooted in our work. We followed a specific structure that allowed for all voices to be heard, and we took time at the end of every meeting to share an appreciation for someone or something from that meeting which helps us to create this continued sense of community building.

In my interview with Lawrence, we reflected on where we put our energy and how we conceptualize art. He stated:

> It's like clowning. It's like a like a play I directed. The King, he's speaking truth to power. It's like the King has all these policies in place, and the clown is making fun of the King, but because he's dressed so funny he doesn't appear to be a threat right? So. But instead, he's actually doing the social movement with the people like acting like the king and acting like a fool, and the people know what he's talking about. King tolerates it because it's like, yeah, well, he's a clown, right? And not to denigrate clowns at all. I mean, that's the true secret of it is that we are in this clown suit, within and within entrepreneurship, or within a capitalistic system, where we are affecting change through the ways that we know how.
>
> I guess from a brown skin point of view, the careful balance is not to get too narrow. Right? Because art is wide and all I can do is bring culture into it, my own culture and use that art to help.

## WIDER AND DEEPER

The work of Art for Social Change has been collaborative, socially conscious, focused on social change, and open to public discourse. Talwar (2016) wrote, "When we locate the therapeutic in social praxis that encourages collective participation, art is no longer an object of contemplation; instead, it becomes a critical and communal process" (p. 846). Our work moved through many cycles of dialogue, action, and reflection, and continues to evolve. The shared ownership and investment of all people have made it what it is. It is our shared values, vision, and reflexive structure that helps us keep a consistent presence and focus over time.

We have embedded structures of support within the graduate art therapy program that are linked directly to this group. Incorporating a public practice art therapy model (Timm-Bottos & Reilly, 2015; Watkins &

Shulman, 2008), we offer an open studio in our new community studio in Portland. This studio is a space for people to process and make art about relevant social, racial, and political events. Students collaborate with Art for Social Change members to develop socially engaged service learning as a part of their training as art therapists, moving theory into action.

Being a social entrepreneur does not necessarily mean creating a new organization. Instead, it involves questioning norms, challenging assumptions, understanding the underlying causes of social issues, and innovatively mobilizing resources to address them. Achieving this requires forming partnerships, fostering interdisciplinary collaboration, and empowering others (Chahine, 2023).

Art for social change embraces a decolonized approach to healing and connection. This work is entrepreneurial, as it emerged out of pain, trauma, disconnection, isolation, and fear. We aligned our shared values and acknowledged that we wanted to create something to address the needs in our community, participating in a collective that was bigger than our individual selves. What we birthed is a space for connection, meaning, reflection, and action that collectively aims toward an anti-oppressive liberatory future.

## REFERENCES


Allen, P. (1992). Artist in residence: An alternative to "clinification" for art therapist. *Art Therapy: Journal of the American Art Therapy Association, 9*(1), 22–29. https://doi.org/10.1080/07421656.1992.10758933

Andrus, M. (2023). Collective storytelling: Art and film to process an unexpected loss. *International Journal of Art Therapy, 28*(4), 187–195. https://doi.org/10.1080/17454832.2023.2188411

Andrus, M., Siulagi, O., & Tsabari, K. (2024). Art for social change: Aligning values and actions toward effective activism. *Art Therapy: Journal of the American Art Therapy Association,* Advance online publication. https://doi.org/10.1080/07421656.2024.2366569

Anzaldúa, G. (1987). *Borderlands/la frontera.* Aunt Lute Books.

Awais, Y. (2022). Naming who performs care: Occupational segregation in the creative arts therapies. *The Arts in Psychotherapy, 80,* Article 101943. https://doi.org/10.1016/j.aip.2022.101943

Awais, Y., & Yali, A. M. (2013). A call for diversity: The need to recruit and retain ethnic minority students in art therapy. *Art Therapy: Journal of the American Art Therapy Association, 30*(3), 130–134. https://doi.org/10.1080/07421656.2013.819284

Bonanno, J. (2018). Capital as the lens that Bourdieu Pierre's through: Public relations, social theory, and rhetoric. *Public Relations Review, 44*(3), 385–392. https://doi.org/10.1016/j.pubrev.2018.04.008

Boston, C., & Short, G. (2011). Notes: Georgette Seabrooke Powell. *Art Therapy: Journal of the American Art Therapy Association, 23*(2), 89–90. https://doi.org/10.1080/07421656.2006.10129649

Bourdieu, P. (1977). *Outline of a theory of practice.* Cambridge University Press.

Brooks, S. (2023, April 19). *Portland perception in decline but still hopeful.* The Oracle: The vision of McDaniel. Retrieved from https://mhsnews.org/1951/opinion/portland-perception-in-decline-but-still-hopeful

brown, a. m. (2017). *Emergent strategies: Shaping change, changing worlds.* AK Press.

Bullard, D. B. (2007). *Academic capitalism in the social sciences: Faculty responses to the entrepreneurial university* [Doctoral dissertation]. University of South Florida, Scholar Commons. Retrieved from https://digitalcommons.usf.edu/etd/647

Caballero, D. (2023, February 1). *Oregon ranks 50th in the US for providing access to addiction treatment: Recovering addicts want better resources.* KGW8. Retrieved from www.kgw.com/article/news/health/oregon-worst-in-nation-for-addiction-treatments-locals-rally-in-salem/283-b2e5b42b-218e-4b2c-9ec5-f3ce9fca8c74#:~:text=Oregon%20currently%20has%20the%20second,in%20providing%20addiction%20treatment%20access

Camhi, T. (2020, June 6). *A racist history shows why Oregon is still so white: Oregon white history racist foundations black exclusion laws.* Oregon Public Broadcasting. Retrieved from www.opb.org/news/article/oregon-white-history-racist-foundations-black-exclusion-laws

Chahine, T. (2023). *Social entrepreneurship: Building impact step by step* (2nd ed.). Routledge.

Doby-Copeland, C. (2019). Intersections of traditional healing and art therapy: Legacy of Sarah E. McGee. *Art Therapy: Journal of the American Art Therapy Association, 36*(3), 157–161. https://doi.org/10.1080/07421656.2019.164954

Dowling, J. (2020, September 8). *Resident says "house filled with tear gas" during riot.* KOIN 6 News. Retrieved from www.koin.com/news/protests/resident-says-house-filled-with-tear-gas-during-riot/#:~:text=PORTLAND%2C%20Ore.,described%20as%20firebombs%20toward%20police

Flaccus, G. (2019, August 17). *At least 13 people arrested at Portland Oregon, protest.* Associated press. Retrieved from https://web.archive.org/web/20201009103452/https://abcnews.go.com/US/wireStory/portland-oregon-awaits-wing-rally-counter-protests-65027584

Freiré, P. (2018). *Pedagogy of the oppressed* (M. Bergman Ramos, Trans.). Bloomsbury.

Gopalakrishna, M. (2022). Practicing in an expanded paradigm: Case examples and ethical anchors for creative arts therapists working in community-based social justice contexts. *The Arts in Psychotherapy, 80,* Article 101921. https://doi.org/10.1016/j.aip.2022.101921

Hayden, N. (2023, April 5). *Oregon's recent growth in homelessness among largest in nation.* Oregon Live: The Oregonian. Retrieved from www.oregonlive.com/politics/2023/04/oregons-recent-growth-in-homelessness-among-largest-in-nation.html#:~:text=Chronic%20homelessness%20has%20been%20quickly,for%20a%20total%20of%206%2C447

hooks, b. (1991). Theory as liberatory practice. *Yale Journal of Law & Feminism, 4*(1/2). Retrieved from http://digitalcommons.law.yale.edu/yjlf/vol4/iss1/2

Howe, A. (2023, June 29). *Supreme Court strikes down affirmative action programs in college admissions.* Scotus Blog. Retrieved from www.scotusblog.com/2023/06/supreme-court-strikes-down-affirmative-action-programs-in-college-admissions

Joseph, C. (1989). Art, politics, and the life force. *Forward: Journal of Socialist Thought, 9*(1), 39–28. Retrieved from https://unityarchiveproject.org/wp-content/uploads/Forward_Vol.9_No.1_Spring_Summer_1989_edit.pdf

Kanerahtenhá:wi Whyte, M., & Toll, H. (2023). Creativity as spirit: Re-indigenization and anticolonialism in art therapy (La créativité en tant qu'esprit: re-indigénisation et anti-colonialisme en art-thérapie). *Canadian Journal of Art Therapy, 36*(1), 2–11. https://doi.org/10.1080/26907240.2023.2213935

Killen, D. (n.d.). *100 days of Portland protests.* Oregon Live: The Oregonian. Retrieved from www.oregonlive.com/galleries/6JTNG23TENDKZBEQ2HW4JPQVP4

Kon, O. (2017, December 18). *Pierre bourdieu: Theory of capital* (social and cultural capital) [Video]. Retrieved from www.youtube.com/watch?v=dQ5MdAjX4NU

Kurtzleben, D. (2020, July 28). *What the "wall of mom's" protests say about motherhood, race in America.* National Public Radio. Retrieved from www.npr.org/2020/07/28/896174019/what-the-wall-of-moms-protests-say-about-motherhood-race-in-america

Lang, M. J. (2020, July 26). *Leaf-blower wars: How Portland protesters are fighting back against tear gas and forming "walls" of veterans, lawyers, and nurses.* The Washington Post. Retrieved from www.washingtonpost.com/nation/2020/07/26/leaf-blower-wars-how-portland-protesters-are-fighting-back-against-tear-gas-forming-walls-veterans-lawyers-nurses

Levinson, J., Wilson, C., Doubek, J., & Nuyen, S. (2020, July 17). *Federal officers use unmarked vehicles to grab people in Portland, DHS confirms.* National Public Radio: All Things Considered. Retrieved from www.npr.org/2020/07/17/892277592/federal-officers-use-unmarked-vehicles-to-grab-protesters-in-portland

Mandler McKnight, C. (2023). Unsettling spirit: A journey into decolonization (Décoloniser les relations, décoloniser l'esprit), by Denise M. Nadeau. *Canadian Journal of Art Therapy, 36*(1), 63–65. https://doi.org/10.1080/26907240.2022.2160547

Martín-Baró, I. (1994). *Writings for a liberation psychology.* Harvard University Press.

McLean, H. (2015). Neoliberalism and the attack on education: An interview with Henry A. Giroux. *Alternate Routes, 26*, 305–311. Retrieved from www.alternateroutes.ca/index.php/ar/article/view/22322

McMillan-Cottom, T. (2017). *Lower ed: The troubling rise of for-profit colleges in the new economy.* The New Press.

Nieto, L., Boyer, M. F., Goodwin, L., Johnson, G. R., & Collier Smith, L. (2010). *Beyond inclusion, beyond empowerment: A developmental strategy to liberate everyone.* Cuetzpalin.

*Ranking the states of 2022.* (n.d.). Mental Health America. Retrieved from https://mhanational.org/issues/2022/ranking-states

Sanders, B. (2023). *It's okay to be angry about capitalism.* Crown.

Şerban, O. (2023). *Cultural capital and creative communication: (Anti-) modern and (non-) eurocentric perspectives.* Routledge.

Stepney, S. A. (2022). Multicultural and diversity perspectives in art therapy: Transforming image into substance. In M. Rastogi, R. P. Feldwisch, M. Pate, & J. Scarce (Eds.), *Foundations of art therapy: Theory and applications* (pp. 79–120). Academic Press.

Talwar, S. (2016). Creating alternative public spaces: Community-based art practice, critical consciousness, and social justice. In D. Gussak & M. Rosal (Eds.), *The Wiley handbook of art therapy* (pp. 840–847). Wiley.

Timm-Bottos, J. (2016). Beyond counseling and psychotherapy, there is a field: I'll meet you there. *Art Therapy: Journal of the American Art Therapy Association, 33*(3), 160–162. https://doi.org/10.1080/07421656.2016.1199248

Timm-Bottos, J., & Reilly, R. C. (2015). Learning in third spaces: Community art studio as storefront university classroom. *American Journal of Community Psychology, 55*(1–2), 102–114. https://doi.org/10.1007/s10464-014-9688-5

Totenberg, N., & McCammon, S. (2022, June 24). *Supreme Court overturns Roe v. Wade, ending right to abortion upheld for decades.* National Public Radio: All Things Considered. Retrieved from www.npr.org/2022/06/24/1102305878/supreme-court-abortion-roe-v-wade-decision-overturn

Trans Legislation Tracker. (n.d.). *Anti-trans bills tracker.* Retrieved from https://trans-legislation.com

U.S. Department of Justice. (2024, September 23). *Federal bureau of investigation: Hate crime Statistics.* Retrieved from www.justice.gov/hatecrimes/hate-crime-statistics

Van Den Berg, Z., & Allen, P. (2022). Specters of whiteness: Radical care for ghostly matters in art therapy. *The Arts in Psychotherapy, 80,* Article 101932. https://doi.org/10.1016/j.aip.2022.101932

Venture, L. D. (1977). *The black beat in art therapy experiences* [Doctoral dissertation]. ProQuest Dissertation and Theses Database. (UMI No. 7720887).

Watkins, M., & Shulman, H. (2008). *Toward psychologies of liberation.* Palgrave Macmillan.

White, M., & Epston, D. (1990). *Narrative means to therapeutic ends.* W. W. Norton.

Wilkerson, I. (2020). *Caste: The origins of our discontents.* Random House.

Wilson, C. (2022, November 29). *Portland agrees to settle 2020 tear gas lawsuit brought by protesters for $250,000.* Oregon Public Broadcasting. Retrieved from www.opb.org/article/2022/11/29/portland-police-protest-oregon-rubber-ball-devices-crowd-control

Wright, T., & Wright, K. (2022). Proposing a justice approach to ethics of care in art psychotherapy. *The Arts in Psychotherapy, 79*(2), 101912. https://doi.org/10.1016/j.aip.2022.101912

Zaitz, L. (2016, January 2). *Militia takes over Malheur National Wildlife Refuge headquarters.* The Oregonian/Oregon Live. Advance Publications. ISSN 8750–1317.

Chapter 4

# The Living Museum, a Contemporary Art Movement

*Mitra Reyhani Ghadim and Rose Ehemann*

In 1983, 40 Creedmoor Psychiatric Center patients walked into an abandoned 40,000 square foot building on the Queens, New York, grounds of Creedmoor. Along with the artist Bolek Greczynski and psychologist Dr. Janos Marton, they began the work of transforming the former kitchen and dining hall into a space for making and exhibiting art (Poser, 2014). This was the initiation of a safe, creative community space.

The Living Museum was an extraordinary concept, an unusual entrepreneurship developed within the state organization. One can think of the Living Museum as a Deleuzian *War Machine* (Deleuze & Guattari, 1986). Philosopher Gilles Deleuze and psychotherapist and philosopher Felix Guattari wrote about a pole of the war machine which seems to be its essence; this is when the war machine with indefinitely lower "quantities" has as its objective not war, but the drawing of a creative line of flight, the composition of a smooth space, and of the movement of people in that space (Deleuze & Guattari, 2009). This was a *war machine* that resisted tree-like forms of growth and centralizing organizational systems. Leaving the striated and controlled roads within communication systems of the state apparatus behind, the founders of the Living Museum took a point of flight from psychiatric hospital systems, developing a new territory. They moved together and created trajectories with patients and later with volunteers, with people who became nomadically de-territorialized from the heavily regulated territories of the state hospital system. They found themselves in a territory where their being, thoughts, works, and creativity could flourish with freedom, where they would safely express themselves. The Living Museum continues to expand its impact globally, and today numerous Living Museums have been established in various cities throughout the world.

DOI: 10.4324/9781032615776-5

At the Living Museums, people spend time by simply *being*, freely, each with their unique relation to the world, and by *becoming*, through freedom for creative work and expressions. The Living Museum was invented as an alternative to commercialism, a fight against commercial art scene models for artists who would be able to work with a specific community and introduce art where it is needed most (Greczynski, 1988).

This chapter unfolds in two sections, both giving the account of arts-based mental health entrepreneurship from the experience of two art therapists, one in New York and another in Wil, Switzerland, each explaining their connections, and their inspirations following their encounter with this extraordinary yet simple creative space, but also conceptual artwork, the Living Museum.

## LIVING MUSEUM, QUEENS VILLAGE, NEW YORK

In this section, Mitra Reyhani Ghadim describes her connection to the first Living Museum of Creedmoor Psychiatric Center in Queens Village, NY, and its ongoing initiatives.

I connected with the Living Museum (LM) as a volunteer artist-in-residence in 2014, while I was undertaking my doctoral studies with professors Dr. Bruce Moon and Dr. Lynn Kapitan at Mount Mary University in Milwaukee, Wisconsin. Several years back, they held an exhibition from the works created by LM artists at Mount Mary University. Noticing my interest in studio-based and museum-based art therapy, Dr. Moon recommended that I connect with Dr. Janos Marton, the co-founder of the LM in New York. At the time, I was leading the Access/Art Therapy program of the Queens Museum of Art (QM) in Queens, New York, full-time, and conducting weekly programs for children and teens with autism spectrum at Nassau County Museum of Art. Because my work schedule included weekends, I started spending my weekday time off at the LM.

At the museum, I was fascinated by the beauty of the day-to-day life of the museum which brings freedom of working on their interest to patient-artists, as well as volunteers. The LM was a utopia, a surreal experience in a grand space where I could make art and socialize with other artists. I was also captivated by the beauty and authenticity of the collections and installations. Working at the LM has been a pleasure; there is no place I would rather be. Every day, I experience joy from discussions with client-artists, museum staff, and volunteers. We talk, exchange ideas, and discuss life, philosophy, politics, art, and cinema. We plan and develop themes for exhibitions and share ideas on other topics, all affecting our thoughts and feelings and our connections with the world.

This nonhierarchical democratic approach at the LM finds its precedent in its history. It reflects the approach established by Bolek Greczynski, the first artist-in-residence of Creedmoor; he was also the co-founder and first director of the LM. When he became associated with Creedmoor, Bolek was an accomplished artist and actor with several conceptual art exhibitions and installations in the United States and internationally. Bolek had a remarkable respect and love for Creedmoor patients. At a time of social stigma for psychiatric diagnoses, he saw patients as friends and colleagues (Yu, 1998). Bolek made a proposal to Creedmoor officials, requesting space to set up an active art workshop and a permanent exhibition space for an ongoing installation produced by the patients (Phillips, 1988). Changing attitudes and legislation concerning long-term hospitalization and the de-institutionalization movement meant Creedmoor's patient population had declined by 400 percent in the previous 15 years, and there were several buildings available. Creedmoor accepted his proposal, and the LM was established (Phillips, 1988). In 1983, Building 75's 40,000 square foot space was transformed into an open art studio where patients could feel empowered, as they no longer would be subjected (only) to labels tied to their mental illness (Queens Museum, 2002).

At that time, the constantly changing artwork and workspace installation was a composition of elements, some planned and others spontaneous, which had a cohesive feel despite its seemingly eclectic assemblage. Patients and Greczynski named their first collaborative project "Battlefields," suggesting the contentiousness of the spaces they inhabited, both psychic and institutional, although the work they produced was the result of fruitful and generous cooperation (Phillips, 1988).

Bolek Greczynski was a remarkable director who developed projects based on issues that were of consequence to patients. He nurtured an open atmosphere for production and experimentation. The original installation in the space was on the second floor, which consisted of a series of rooms and a caged corridor overlooking the former kitchen, in a square configuration wrapped around a large central atrium. The four corner room installations each had a theme: *hospital, church, workplace,* and *home sweet home.* Objects and furniture from the old dining hall were incorporated into the art (Phillips, 1988).

During the early months of my weekly visits to the museum in 2014, I had noticed that group visitors to the museum are almost exclusively medical, psychiatry, and psychology students who came to see the space and the art of people with mental illness. This was a good learning opportunity for them, but I wanted to develop a project where LM artists would be invited to join a monthly open studio at the Queens Museum (QM), to be exposed to other community activities. The LM had a history of collaboration with the QM, going back to 2003, when the LM exhibition

*In the Flow* was hosted at Queens Museum (QM). *In the Flow* celebrated art that was controversial, which as a result existed on the periphery of the art world (Marton et al., 2002). In 2014, my wish was to create lateral connections between the LM and QM studio spaces. I wanted to initiate fluid movements that would bring artists of the LM to the QM galleries and studios, to make art, and to visit contemporary art exhibitions, and be in a space beyond the outpatient campus grounds. I believed that with these nomadic movements for deterritorialization, the artists of LM could experience contemporary art exhibits in QM galleries, as well as be in a new space to meet people, families, and visitors of the contemporary museum. This two-way connection brought the opportunity for LM artists to make new connections with other communities outside of Creedmoor Psychiatric grounds. Their art and thoughts would be shared with others in a different context. I later curated an exhibit of 14 artists from the LM artists at Hofstra University, where we had the artists speak about their work and interact with students and faculty.

After a change in leadership at the QM significantly impacted education programs, decreasing their scope and vibrance, I joined the New York State Office of Mental Health (NYS OMH) Sagamore Children's Center in 2019. Sagamore is an inpatient long-term hospital for children ages 6–17, located in Dix Hills, NY. There, I started the creative arts department, and I established a small children's LM in an underutilized space. Two years later, as Creedmoor Psychiatric Center's LM was in search of a new director, they notified me, and I transferred to work at Creedmoor Psychiatric Center's LM.

Dr. Janos Marton has been a mentor and valuable friend to me since I connected with the museum a decade ago. My current work as director is informed by his teaching, particularly by his positive energy, curiosity, creative thinking, kindness, empathy, and love for people, animals, nature. Since starting at the LM, I have been organizing the existing artworks and documents, and an impressive number of photos of patient-artists and volunteers who have formed the creative force behind the museum since 1983. Those patient-artists and volunteers (featured in in hundreds of photos) as well as those who are involved with the museum today can be described with the well-known slogan of German artist Joseph Beuys who said "Everyone is an artist," suggesting that social transformation can be achieved if every human being applied their creative energies toward positive change in cooperative activities he called *Social Sculpture* (Walker Art Center, 2024).

Creedmoor Psychiatric Center is the largest psychiatric facility in New York City. It was the first hospital in the United States to systematically collect and produce art by people with mental illness (Marton et al., 2002). Today, the LM holds the largest collection of art by client-artists with mental illness in the United States (and likely globally). This collection must be archived and shared with others. Taking over such a large space, collection, and concept, and creating new ideas, has been intimidating but also exciting. My decade at the QM had prepared me for leadership and management, and working at Sagamore Children's Center (as well as previous work at Mount Sinai Hospital's adult behavioral unit) prepared me for aspects of the work pertaining to psychiatric hospitals. At the QM, I admired the thinking and the approach of then-executive director Tom Finkelpearl, who gave museum staff the autonomy to practice and implement what we were passionate about: he believed in our vision. I successfully applied this approach to my work at the QM. At the QM, every project was either developed or assigned to a person who would take on special ownership due to their interest and passion for a particular type of project.

When I started as director of the LM, I knew the museum would shift from being open four days a week to five days, and that it would no longer be managed by one staff plus volunteers. I selected staff with a mindset aligned with art and creative work from the hospital's other departments and I currently work with two full-time staff. The LM is part of the state grounds and is surrounded by nature. My art therapist colleague Patricia Vehrum, who has a passion for gardening, and I decided to take advantage of the LM's grounds and developed an outdoor gardening and indoor horticulture areas. We transformed one of the museum's rooms into a space for horticulture and added a greenhouse to the outdoor garden so we could extend gardening into cooler months. For the past two years, artists have engaged in gardening projects and learned about healthy food while enjoying organic vegetables directly from our garden. At times we prepare food using these vegetables and enjoy a communal lunch together. Seeing other colleagues' interests, I added writing and journaling, dance, music ensemble, and a film club. I brought back the Tai Chi class (which had previously been offered and discontinued), and later increased its sessions due to general interest. We added an English as a Second Language class. Most recently, building on an area of interest of my colleague, rehabilitation counselor Brienne Johnson (LMHC, CASAC), we started a mosaic art workshop.

Reflecting on the history and the artwork accumulated during the last four decades, we decided to create artwork for a show in the museum space about the concept of time (Figure 4.1). We had an opening reception in November 2023, and artists continue to make contributions to the exhibit; we will have a culminating event in the spring.

With an interest in bringing artists to the museum, I established affiliations with Long Island University, Pratt Institute, and NYU. We have one to three student interns each semester, who bring additional interest and passions, and who make contributions to this arts-based community.

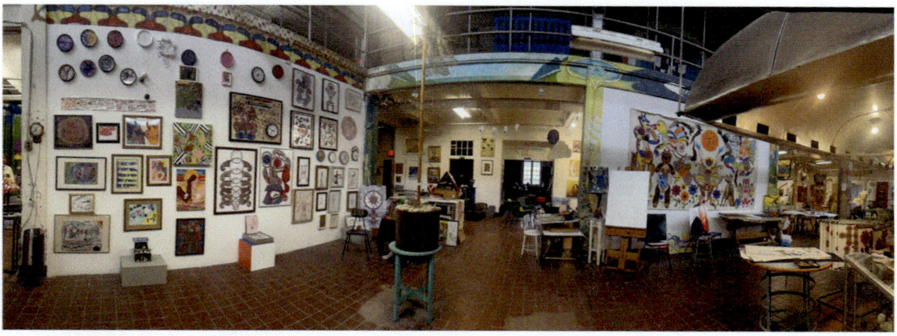

***Figure 4.1*** *Time Exhibit.*

*Note*: The center space of the Living Museum NY during the 2023–2024 exhibition, "Time." Photograph taken by Mitra Reyhani Ghadim.

The LM has had numerous volunteers and visitors since its founding, from across the United States and internationally, some of whom developed LMs in their own towns and countries, either as stand-alone organizations or within their place of work. In the Unites States, art therapist Christine Randolph developed the Rockland County LM (RLM) in 2010. RLM is a studio that serves a community of artists who are inpatient or outpatient clients at Rockland Psychiatric Center in Orangeburg, New York (Randolph, 2019). "When artists attend the RLM for the first time, they are surprised by the level of freedom that exists in a democratic and voluntary studio" (Randolph, 2019, p. 233), which reflects a common characteristic of LMs' philosophy.

## LIVING MUSEUM, WIL, SWITZERLAND

In this section, I, Rose Ehemann, describe my initial connection with the LM in Queens, New York, and the subsequent growth and expansion of LMs outside of the United States.

During my studies of art therapy at the University of Cologne, in Germany, my professor organized an excursion to New York to visit important art therapy pioneers, such as Edith Kramer at New York University and Arthur Robbins at Pratt Institute. We also visited the LM, in Queens, New York. While in the creative space of the LM, I could not believe that something like that would be possible. Freedom for everybody. No rules dictate what you have to do. Just inspiration, warmth, and authentic artists with mental illness running the place and teaching you many essential things about life. I decided to apply to volunteer at the LM to learn more about their philosophy from Dr. Janos Marton, one of the LM's founders. He has continued to teach me so much, even after my time as intern. We have stayed connected throughout the years, and remain both a mentor and supervisor.

The LM concept is seen as a significant contribution to tackling the increasing prevalence of mental illness, even in times of healthcare staff shortages and rising costs. It is an innovative project, celebrating the diversity of people with mental illness and bringing meaning into their lives. By creating a community of like-minded people and promoting recovery through art, the LM supports psychological stability, reduces hospitalization, reduces stigma, enables positive identity transformation and suicide prevention, and thus also closes gaps in psychiatric care. In addition, the LM is an art movement itself, as everybody involved is creating social utopia, artwork, and visions which add to an ever-changing art performance. Each art piece and person continues to add to an expansive international social sculpture with the potential to transform society. Like a successful art movement, it has been multiplying fast at an international level, as the philosophy it holds is universally understood and appreciated. There is a strong connection among LM founders and directors.

Back in Europe, after completing my studies in art therapy, I first held a job as an art educator working with teenagers in Berlin. After two years, we turned the youth residence into an art space, and we created an art magazine. In 2002, after moving to Switzerland, I had to restart my professional life. I wrote to various clinics, offering speeches and presentations about the Living Museum of New York, with the idea of implementing the LM in a psychiatric institution in Switzerland. Psychiatric University Clinic in Zurich invited me for a lecture; the philosophy impressed the audience. Later I was invited to a job interview at the psychiatric clinic in Wil where I took the opportunity to talk with the chief of psychiatry about the LM, which proved to be a great opportunity. He immediately understood the impact this could have on patients and, more importantly, on the image of the clinic. He told the head of nursing in Wil, near St. Gallen, to hire me and give me freedom to establish the LM in their psychiatric clinic, which was a wonderful opportunity.

Initially, I was provided a 250 square meter (about 2,700 sq. ft.) room where I was able to start creating art with patients and work on their identity change from mental patients to artists. Since that time in 2002, we have become the second LM in the world. Slowly I implemented the philosophy, tried to adjust to the existing structure of the hospital system, which meant becoming familiar with the personnel, the technology, how the processes of psychiatric treatments in this clinic were structured, and how patients could take part in programs. A flyer was created to inform hospital patients and staff about the start of the LM and about the procedures for patient participation. It was sent to each ward and the day clinic. Soon the treatment teams on the wards sent patients to the LM. I prepared an in-service presentation and an exhibition to disseminate the information among the employees of the psychiatric clinic, including doctors, psychologists, nurses, social workers, and other therapists. Some staff were critical; they thought that one cannot give the patients so much freedom, that one needs more control over them, and one should not show their artwork in public. While running the LM, I expanded my professional training, studied arts management, and I completed my doctorate in art therapy in 2014. The skills in arts management helped me in organizing large-scale international exhibitions and managing the roll-out of more LMs in Switzerland and Europe. My doctoral thesis required meticulous scientific work, and my mentor, Prof. Dr. Barbara Wichelhaus, taught me scientific discipline and precision. My doctorate convinced science-oriented mental health professionals of the reliability and the seriousness of my ambitions in establishing more LMs and gave me access to these circles.

After few years, the management staff of the clinic were convinced of the tremendous impact of the LM and invited us to expand, so that the LM could move into a 700 square meter building (about 7,600 sq. ft.) with space for a beautiful outdoor garden. I later inquired to find out how many other creative therapists might already among the 750 employees of this large clinic; I thought perhaps I could inspire them to collaborate with me in different art projects and exhibitions. There was an existing ceramic studio, first run by a ceramic artist and then by artist and art psychotherapist Nicole Ottiger, who accepted my request to be responsible for the management of the LM. There was also a paper studio run by two creative therapists and a work studio run by a design teacher. Following these connections and collaborations, we were allowed to expand again and could all move together to a three-story 2000 square meter (about 22,000 sq. ft.) building. Here we established six different art studios, each dedicated to a different medium: digital media arts, ceramics, music, theater, glass, wood, and paper. After developing these programs within the new building, I convinced the leadership of the clinic to hire landscape therapist Berndt Vogel to apply the LM philosophy to the outdoor area as a nature studio and allow us to do artwork with and within nature, as well as work with animals. He joined us, and within a few years, he transformed the entire outside space of the clinic into a LM where visitors could make tours through the beautiful grounds.

In 2012, our LM was invited to collaborate with Heimstätten Wil, which is a day center for people with mental illness, and is located on the same grounds as the psychiatric clinic. Because of the broad network I developed and my many years of experience, I was invited during the planning phase to help with defining the structure, setting, and expansion of the day center. This opportunity helped LM Wil to not only expand in size, with more clients and staff involved, but also allowed people with chronic mental illness to stay long-term and lifelong at the LM, should they need it.

I was invited to work 10% as an art coach and supervisor for the day center which was directed by Cornelia Christen and 90% as the director of the LM of the psychiatric clinic. I took the opportunity because it allowed people with chronic illness to stay in residential facilities of the LM Wil; they did not have to leave after treatment in clinic had ended. The LM initiative grew into a large art movement within the psychiatric grounds. The patients connect with each other and build a caring LM artist community. The LM is run mainly by the patients themselves, providing peer support essential for their psychic stabilization. The change of identity leads to recovery, because for the first time in their lives they are seen with their great artistic potential. The art that comes out of the LM spreads out over the whole grounds of the psychiatric clinic. Employees choose artwork from our artists for their offices and the art enlightens all public spaces. Art is now everywhere on the grounds.

## INTERNATIONAL EXPANSION OF LMs

As mentioned earlier, I completed a degree in arts management at the University of Basel. This training allowed me to deepen my abilities as a presenter while I gained knowledge and skills that prepared me for a diverse range of responsibilities in management, arts administration, entrepreneurship, arts education, cultural policy and advocacy, and arts philanthropy. It also enabled me to manage large-scale international art projects.

The first volunteer of the LM Wil, Magdalena Steinemann, had the dream to establish another LM in Winterthur in Switzerland. To be able to raise money, we had to establish a nonprofit organization, and we founded the Living Museum Society Switzerland in 2012. We had to learn so much about leading a nonprofit organization, about the structure, the legal aspects, and much more. Some of the main skills needed for a successful nonprofit are strategic planning, financial management, fundraising, marketing and communication, leadership and decision-making, organizational development, and volunteer management. Both my training and my former engagement as president of the Confederation of Swiss Art Therapy Associations (gpk) in Switzerland helped me gain skills in leading a nonprofit organization. We were also comparing the structures of various other nonprofit organizations to adapt them to the new community where these were going to be established. The mission of the association has been to spread the LM philosophy and help others in the process of building LMs in Switzerland, Europe, and the world.

Due to the nonprofit organization and successful fundraising, the board of The Living Museum Society Switzerland was able to help to establish ten more LMs in Switzerland: Zurich, Bern, Lichtensteig, Münsingen, Solothurn, Rorschach, Kreuzlingen, Schaffhausen, Ticino, and Basel and they are about to open even more in the year 2024. The LM Madrid, in Spain, already started, and in Germany the LM Alb, which was the first, and Potsdam have launched. There is also the potential to help to start more LMs in Spain, France, Austria (LM Linz), Italy, Bulgaria, Ukraine, and Germany (LM Munich). Expansion will also include five more LMs in Germany and five in additional countries.

Besides the work of this nonprofit organization, other projects have been developed. Four LMs have been founded in the Netherlands since 2015, with the initiative of Rokus Lopik. Jennifer Hyojin Lee, who trained in New York, started a LM in 2017 in Seoul, South Korea; Natia Pandjikidze started one in Tbilisi, Georgia, and Alexandra Plettenberg, a previous longtime volunteer at the LM New York, will start a LM in Graz, Austria.

Some founders developed living museums independent from any institutions, which comes with the risk of not being able to source enough money for the rents, salaries, and other expenses. To succeed, one has to work hard, dedicate at least one full day per week to connect with philanthropists, foundations, and other supporters to raise funds and to maintain the network. The LM Lyss had to close after two years because the founders retired and could not find a person to take it over as there was no sustainable financing. Luckily, we were able to transport the whole infrastructure to the LM Alb in South Germany, which had just opened at that time.

What helped in the process of spreading LMs was to talk about it at any opportunity. Presentations and articles helped in the process of making the philosophy more well known. We invited teams from different organizations to do team-building events at the LM. We networked in the sectors of mental health and art, because LMs can be located at the interface between the two disciplines. Now we are even connected with the World Health Organization and the UN. Both help us to spread the philosophy in countries we cannot easily access. There is a Social Prescribing movement at the World Health Organization that will hopefully integrate the LM in their catalog (WHO Team, 2022). Isabelle Wachsmuth, responsible for art impact for health at the World Health Organization and UN, is preparing for that initiative. Angela Samata from Liverpool (who was awarded the Winston Churchill fellowship and conducted research in LMs) is helping in the international scaling of LMs. What also helped in the scaling of the LM as a model was the foundation of the International LM Academy. Nicole Ottiger has finished her doctorate and together we were able to establish the program to educate interested persons from art and mental health professions in the LM philosophy. We teach how to build up and run an LM and involve them in the international network. If they complete the academy, the trainees receive the title and certificate "International LM Director."

We hire as staff artists doing their own professional artwork who are interested in working with an artist community. They must know how to prepare, organize, and curate exhibitions. They must be open and flexible personalities with empathy and kindness. Reliability and nonjudgmental attitude are important strengths we look for. The willingness to serve other people and to treat them with equal rights is also a desired skill. As a leader, one should have the ability to create vision, empower people, delegate, and lead with a participatory approach. Success also comes through the creativity of the staff, the visions they create and realize together. A free environment where all are allowed to learn and grow is very important.

Business skills are needed to start an independent project. It is essential to cultivate networking abilities and develop cross-cultural communication and collaboration skills for finding supporting partners. It is important to have a "serendipity mindset," which allows one to connect persons and situations and find the right time for certain challenges. Most importantly, one must have passion, so that they remain steady and resilient in following their vision.

Staying connected with the network of founders was very helpful in scaling the model of the LM. Also, connecting with people with knowledge of the health sector, the art sector, and the finance sector who are committed to being on the board of our association. We asked another nonprofit organization, "Innovage," a group of retired entrepreneurs who coach other nonprofit organizations for only a small fee. They always helped in preparing business plans, gave access to their networks and engaged more than expected in coaching the single projects in different cities. The exchanges within the community of practice of the international LM Directors' remote meetings are very supportive and allow learning from each other, helping each other, and growing together as a community. We are successful with the organization because we are so convinced about the impact of the project on our society as a whole. We put in as much time as possible, because it is a lot of fun and full of meaning. This drives and motivates us.

In the future, we aim to establish an international Living Museum Foundation, a global umbrella organization that functions as an international network for LMs and promotes the exchange of knowledge, networking, and the further development of the LM movement. To support and connect these expanding community networks in various countries, a Founders' Wiki will be built by this community of practice to provide easy access to all important concepts, business plans, corporate identity material and more.

## FINAL NOTES

As art therapists, teaching artists, and mental health professionals, we continue to develop structures and spaces where people can create more territories that reflect diverse realities and make these more visible to society at large (Dejkameh & Sabbaghi, 2019). The LM is a sustainable movement because of its adaptability, which allows its development worldwide, through the initiative and passion of its leaders and their teams. A common tenet of LMs as joyful and peaceful places holds that, aside from basic expectations about respecting each other and protecting everyone's safety, there are no rules, no right or wrong, no good or bad, and there is support for artist-clients, but no judgment (Randolph, 2019). It is our hope that this movement will reach many places in the world, including countries and cities with fewer resources, especially areas affected by war, migrations and displacement, poverty, and addiction, to support people experiencing challenges by being third spaces, and territories for positive impacts on the well-being of communities.

## REFERENCES


Dejkameh, M., & Sabbaghi, V. (2019). From *Please Touch* to Art *Access*: A rhizomatic growth. In A. Wexler & V. Sabbaghi (Eds.), *Bridging communities through socially engaged art* (1st ed., pp. 57–66). Routledge.

Deleuze, G., & Guattari, F. (1986). *Nomadology: The war machine.* Semiotext.

Deleuze, G., & Guattari, F. (2009). *Anti Oedipus: Capitalism and schizophrenia.* Penguin Classics.

Greczynski, B. (1988). *Project description letter.* Queens Village, New York; The Living Museum.

Marton, J., Queens Museum of Art, & Creedmoor Psychiatric Center. (2002). *In the flow: Artists from the living museum: Queens Museum of Art, March 10–July 7, 2002.* New York: Queens Museum of Art.

Phillips, P. C. (1988). Bolek greczynski and the people of the creedmoor psychiatric center, "battlefields" the living museum, creedmoor psychiatric center. *ArtForum, 26*(5). Retrieved from www.artforum.com/events/bolek-greczynski-and-the-people-of-the-creedmoor-psychiatric-center-battlefields-221852/

Poser, S. (2014). *Id-Ego-Superego, art from the living museum at creedmoor psychiatric center.* New York: Center for Modern Psychoanalytic Studies.

Queens Museum. (2002). *Queens Museum: In the flow: Artists from the living museum.* Queens Museum | In the Flow: Artists from the Living Museum. Retrieved from https://queensmuseum.org/exhibition/in-the-flow/

Randolph, C. (2019). The rockland living museum, an open art studio in a psychiatric hospital. In A. Wexler & V. Sabbaghi (Eds.), *Bridging communities through socially engaged art* (1st ed., pp. 233–239). Routledge.

Walker Art Center. (2024). *Joseph Beuys* [Artist Page]. Walker Art Center. Retrieved from http://walkerart.org/collections/artists/joseph-beuys

WHO Team. (2022). *A toolkit on how to implement social prescribing.* World Health Organization. Retrieved from www.who.int/publications/i/item/9789290619765

Yu, J. (Director). (1998). *The living museum* [Film]. HBO, Living Filmworks.

Chapter 5

# Healing Work Is Justice Work

## The Development and Marketing of Art Therapy Services Using an Intersectionality Framework

*Chandra Davis*

In 2007, I began working as an art therapist at a psychiatric hospital in the Greater Washington, D.C. area, focusing on individuals with a history of childhood abuse and neglect. While our unit served as a beacon of hope for those navigating crises and childhood traumas, I observed a significant underrepresentation of marginalized communities in therapy. Marginalized communities such as racial and ethnic minorities, lesbian, gay, bisexual, transgender, queer, questioning, intersex, asexual, plus individuals, and low-income population, often face systemic barriers to accessing mental health services, including art therapy. These barriers, or mental health disparities, can derive from differences in the access to care, quality of care, prevalence of, and outcomes related to mental health conditions among various communities (Cook et al., 2007; Williams et al., 2019).

In a striking example, a Chinese American woman admitted to the psychiatric unit shared her experiences of childhood neglect and physical abuse from her parents, receiving empathetic responses from fellow patients. However, when she revealed her family's connection to the "Chinese Mafia" and its impact on her working-class Chinese immigrant community, the group reacted differently, dismissing her claims as lies and inappropriate for discussion. This stark contrast in responses showcased the challenges of addressing intersectional identity in contrast to more conventional narratives of childhood abuse.

As I delved deeper into my work, I encountered widening mental health disparities that systematically isolated marginalized individuals from receiving appropriate therapy. Addressing the nuances of intersectional identity required a departure from conventional narratives surrounding childhood abuse and trauma, which often failed to fully account for the complexities facing these communities. In 2014, I realized that establishing a private

DOI: 10.4324/9781032615776-6

practice would allow me to work more directly with clients who shared my identities, shaping the messaging and mission of my practice with my desire to support the needs of marginalized populations. The journey, however, was not without obstacles. As I distanced myself from established systems to build this new framework, I became acutely aware of the difficulties in initiating change within an environment that many of my professional peers did not recognize as fundamentally inequitable. Rushin's poem, *The Bridge*, deeply resonated with me during this transition:

> The bridge I must be
> Is the bridge to my own power
> I must translate
> My own fears
> Mediate
> My own weaknesses
> I must be the bridge to nowhere
> But my true self
> And then
> I will be useful
> (Rushin, 2015, pp. xxxiii–xxxiv)

These words reminded me that before I could truly advocate for change, I had to first bridge the gap within myself—between my fears and my purpose, between my doubts and my drive to create a more inclusive art therapy space.

In this chapter, I illustrate how specific marketing strategies can address disparities by reaching marginalized communities, fostering diversity in the client base, and creating a sustainable business that reflects cultural humility, promotes equity, and recognizes systemic oppression in mental health. In addition, I describe how intersectionality is a relevant theoretical framework within art therapy, an idea which has been proposed by many notable art therapists and art therapy scholars for many years (see Datlen & Pandolfi, 2020; Eastwood et al., 2023; Gipson, 2015; Karcher, 2017; Talwar, 2010; Talwar & Sajnani, 2022; Wright & Wright, 2017; Zappa, 2017). Finally, I discuss the ways in which I used an intersectionality framework as a multifaceted approach for marketing my own practice and services, attracting clients seeking inclusive therapeutic spaces and establishing my role as a community advocate and partner.

## AT THE FOUNDATION: INTERSECTIONALITY AS THEORY AND PRACTICE

"Intersectionality," a term coined by Kimberlee Crenshaw (1989), and developed by feminist scholars like Claudia Jones, bell hooks, and Cherrie

Moraga, played a vital role in advancing social justice movements led by women of color, addressing colonialism, racism, and sexism. In her paper *Demarginalizing the Intersection of Race and Sex*, Crenshaw (1989) introduced the concept of intersectionality, highlighting how overlapping factors like race, gender, age, and sexuality shape individuals' experiences of discrimination. Her work, particularly focused on Black women, exposed the deep-seated impacts of patriarchy, white supremacy, capitalism, and other systemic forces on their lives (Collins & Bilge, 2016).

The Oxford English Dictionary (2013) defines "intersectionality" as the interconnected nature of social categorizations like race, class, and gender, creating overlapping systems of discrimination or disadvantage Today, intersectionality acknowledges that everyone's experiences of discrimination and oppression are unique and multifaceted, encompassing factors like gender, race, class, sexual orientation, and physical ability. In essence, intersectionality recognizes that all forms of oppression are interconnected.

Critics argue that intersectionality can be overly complex and challenging to apply practically (Crenshaw, 1991). Some believe it may inadvertently foster victimhood or divisiveness among identity groups, hindering social cohesion (Tomlinson, 2013). However, intersectionality highlights the multifaceted nature of identities shaped by socio-historical, political, and psychological factors, influencing social roles and mental well-being. Understanding intersectionality fosters awareness of disparities faced by marginalized communities and the importance of seeking mental health services, shedding light on the disparities these communities endure.

## ART THERAPIST AS SOCIAL JUSTICE ENTREPRENEUR

As a Black woman art therapist, my work is grounded in intersectionality. My journey of understanding my intersecting identities—Black, woman, art therapist, entrepreneur—revealed the profound impact of seeing other women of color represented in the field of art therapy, a validation that was essential to my growth and sense of belonging. This representation underscored the importance of empowering clients through visibility, acknowledging that, like me, they benefit from seeing themselves reflected in spaces dedicated to their healing. As I learned more about intersectionality theory and developed a more intimate relationship with my intersectional identities—being a Black, woman, art therapist, entrepreneur, etc.—I began to see how intersectionality could be used as a bridge for mending mental health disparities for marginalized communities. As well as how it can be used to examine the various factors that contribute to these disparities. Consideration of these factors helped me to create effective strategies for marketing my business to marginalized communities by prioritizing inclusivity, cultural humility, and empowerment.

Marketing art therapy services is akin to building a bridge connecting therapists and their target audience, establishing a firm foundation for a thriving business. Marketing enables art therapist entrepreneurs to connect with their desired clientele, cultivate a loyal client base, and establish a sustainable business. Intersectionality emerges as a potent and ethical marketing strategy in this endeavor. By acknowledging and addressing the multifaceted identities and experiences of prospective clients, art therapists can construct a bridge that promotes trust and engagement, that is achieved by culturally tailoring community outreach, forging collaborations and partnerships, and harnessing resources like social media to align marketing efforts effectively.

Although specific research on art therapy marketing is limited, the positive impact of marketing on service engagement is undeniable. This opens a door for art therapists to embrace their role as social justice entrepreneurs. By leveraging intersectionality, they can bridge the gap and connect with marginalized communities. Here are some strategies they can use.

## Strategies for Marketing for Connection With Marginalized Communities

*Client outreach through cultural humility training and intersectional workshops*: Continuously educating yourself about cultural humility and the specific needs of different communities demonstrates a commitment to ongoing learning.

Moreover, integrating this knowledge into specialized training programs for art therapists, like implicit bias training, equips therapists to deliver more intersectional care. Art therapists can further extend their impact by organizing workshops or support groups specifically designed to address issues of intersectionality and empowerment within marginalized communities, providing a space for communal healing (Paine et al., 2018).

*Supervision and peer support to unlearn explicit and implicit biases*: Art therapists, like many professionals, can work to address and reduce both explicit and implicit biases in their practice. The ethical standards provided by the Art Therapy Credentials Board (2021) state that art therapists must maintain high standards of professional competence and integrity. Through education, training, and experience, art therapists can develop and improve multicultural competence and cultural humility to provide more effective care. In addition, clinicians must be mindful of countertransference and how it may be influenced by biases or unresolved issues. Regular supervision with experienced, board-certified art therapists and peer support groups can provide a safe space for art therapists to discuss their biases, challenges, and growth in their practice (Wilson et al., 1984). We *all* have implicit bias and reducing one's implicit bias should include an exploration of one's own culture and how it may influence our perceptions and interactions (American Psychological Association, 2023).

*Establishing credibility with culturally responsive messaging and inclusive imagery and language:* Craft marketing materials that acknowledge the unique challenges and experiences of individuals with diverse backgrounds, using inclusive language to signal your business's welcoming attitude to all (American Psychological Association, 2023). It is equally important to include diverse imagery, visually representing your commitment to diversity and inclusivity (American Psychological Association, 2017). Featuring a wide range of people through inclusive imagery sends a powerful message about your commitment to diversity. It strengthens your marketing efforts while showing your qualifications, experience, and ethical commitment.

*Social media and digital engagement as an educational tool:* Marketing provides an opportunity to educate the public about the benefits of art therapy. Through blog posts, workshops, and social media content, art therapists can disseminate information about mental health and healing. They can maintain an active social media presence that promotes social justice, diversity, and inclusivity, sharing content that resonates with marginalized communities (APA, 2017). However, it is important to note that social media is not without its challenges, including issues like online harassment, echo chambers, and misinformation. While social media has the potential to be inclusive and empowering, it can also be a platform for hate and discrimination. Therefore, creating a truly inclusive and equitable online environment requires continuous efforts to address these challenges and promote respectful and constructive dialogue (Imran, 2022).

*Tailoring services to a more client-centered approach:* Highlight your commitment to a client-centered approach, where therapy is tailored to everyone's intersecting identities and experiences (Paine et al., 2018). Inspired by Carl Roger's (1957) person-centered therapy, therapists using these techniques establish a strong connection with their clients' unique needs and experiences. To address economic disparities, offering sliding scale fees can make art therapy accessible for individuals with limited financial resources (Malchiodi, 2018). This practice becomes even more impactful when engaging with clients who embody intersecting identities, as it respects each person's unique lived experiences. By pairing inclusive art therapy techniques with accessible pricing, practitioners can encourage the sharing of diverse narratives, fostering a more compassionate and interconnected community.

*Building a client base by offering sliding scale fees:* Successful marketing efforts aimed at assisting clients from economically disadvantaged backgrounds through a sliding scale fee require a multifaceted approach that emphasizes accessibility, empathy, and community engagement (Practice Solutions, 2016). Leveraging social media platforms, targeted advertising, and community outreach initiatives can effectively raise awareness of the sliding scale fee option among potential clients.

*Community engagement to help destigmatizing mental health:* Actively engage with communities through local events, workshops, or partnerships, demonstrating your dedication to being a part of these communities (American Psychological Association, 2017). Collaborating with local community organizations, such as community centers or nonprofits, can further extend reach and credibility, positioning the art therapist and/or practice as a trusted resource within the community. By implementing and crafting messaging that emphasizes inclusivity, accessibility, and empathy, the art therapist's practice can effectively reach and support clients from disadvantaged backgrounds, contributing to greater equity in mental healthcare access.

*Cultivate and promote liberation-based healing:* Liberation-based healing is a therapeutic practice that centers on the empowerment and liberation of individuals from systemic and personal forms of oppression, trauma, and suffering (Almeida & Tubbs, 2020). Rooted in social justice principles, it acknowledges the impact of societal inequalities and seeks to address them as part of the healing process. By creating a safe and inclusive space for clients to explore their experiences through artistic expression, art therapists can help clients reclaim their narratives and foster self-empowerment and agency (Shafir et al., 2020). Art therapists can infuse techniques such as narrative therapy, mindfulness, and trauma-informed elements into their practice to address the specific needs of individuals and create social change in communities.

*Leveraging Entrepreneurship to Champion Mental Health and Community Advocacy:* As an entrepreneur and business owner, leverage your platform to promote mental health awareness, actively challenge systemic barriers that impact marginalized communities, and provide accessible resources and information. By using your voice and influence, you can foster a culture of support and inclusion, ensuring that mental health becomes a priority for all, especially those facing inequities. Through marketing efforts that share educational content and highlight the transformative potential of art therapy, art therapists can champion mental health policy changes and raise awareness on a broader scale. Promoting inclusive therapeutic spaces provides art therapists with unique opportunities to solidify their positions as community advocates and partners, offering valuable support to individuals and the broader community.

Embracing intersectionality in marketing, art therapists can become social justice entrepreneurs addressing disparities in marginalized communities. This approach attracts clients and promotes equity in mental healthcare. Nevertheless, these endeavors come with significant challenges, including burnout and other emotional tolls from addressing deeply rooted societal issues and taking reputational risks in opposing voices in the community. In the following section, I discuss how I applied intersectionality to align my work as an art therapist with my values, effectively reaching marginalized communities, and fostering communal healing while navigating associated risks.

## COMMUNITY OUTREACH THROUGH CULTURAL HUMILITY: THE BRIDGE COMMUNAL HEALING GROUP

Informed by Kimberlee Crenshaw's work on intersectionality (1991), I co-facilitated The Bridge, a community-healing group. The group offered process therapy sessions for Black women to explore the intersections of their race, gender, and intergenerational trauma. A process therapy group is a guided setting for individuals to explore and share thoughts and experiences, focusing on dynamic interactions for personal growth under the guidance of a trained therapist. In group discussions, we tackled a range of topics, from debunking stereotypes to using art therapy to explore and celebrate the multifaceted nature of intersectionality in their lived experiences.

The name of the communal healing group, The Bridge, drew inspiration from Donna Kate Rushin's *The Bridge Poem* (Rushin, 2015). The bridge serves as a metaphor, symbolizing one's journey, growth, connections, and transition from one place to another. In her poem, Rushin employs the metaphor of bridges to illustrate the role of a Black woman as a bridge to her parents, peers, society, and herself (1981). The various roles described in the poem mirror intersectionality, as Rushin vividly portrays, navigating the complexities of being Black and a woman, grappling with prioritization challenges in different contexts.

Building on the principles of intersectionality previously discussed, my work as a Black woman art therapist involves collaborating with fellow Black women to address race, gender, and intergenerational trauma through a healing approach that empowers individuals and views healing as a collective, transformative process aimed at dismantling systemic inequalities and fostering social justice. Like a bridge connecting landmasses, it unites diverse facets of each person's identity, using Crenshaw's concept as a sturdy framework. During group sessions, the participating women represent their bridges through art. The art-making process and resulting artwork facilitate a dialogue among participants, collectively addressing their challenges.

As I guide others in exploring their identities, I am constantly reflecting on my own intersectional identities, acknowledging how they shape my experiences and practice. The group's courage and vulnerability in sharing

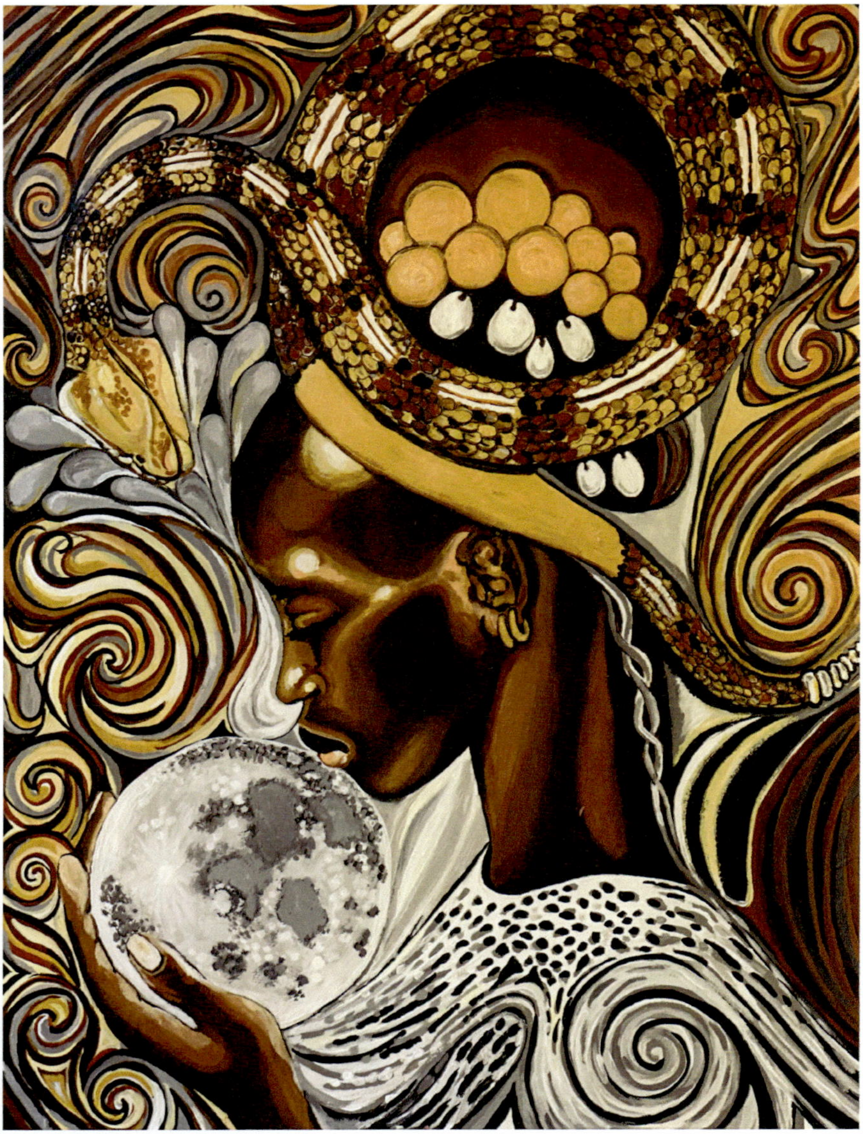

***Figure 5.1*** *"Bridging the Moon, Birthing the Sun" by Chandra Davis.*

*Note*: Response art to the Black women's communal healing group, honoring their rich intersectional identities and acknowledging the profound experiences of feminine and maternal bonds.

their stories deeply inspires me, and prompted me to create a painting that symbolizes my own identities (Figure 5.1). Through this personal artistic expression, I honor the interconnectedness of my identity as a Black woman, art therapist, and advocate for social justice, bridging together my experiences into a visual narrative that stands alongside those of the women I work with.

We began the first session with a liberation-based art therapy exercise, using a metaphorical bridge to guide women participating in the group to their true selves. This process involved exploring their current state, acknowledging layers of identity, and using art to visualize a journey toward self-liberation and their authentic selves. The art exercise offered a creative therapeutic space for them to explore personal narratives, confront obstacles, and embark on a path toward self-liberation.

The women in the bridge group, through art, vividly expressed the significance of their intersectional identities in the healing process. Intersectionality forms the basis for decolonizing mental health clinical practice. Unlike traditional Western psychological paradigms, it addresses the need for systemic change. Trauma-informed care focuses on trauma but often neglects identities of resistance and resourcefulness within a broader systemic context (Ginwright, 2018). An intersectional approach moves away from a siloed framework, recognizing the overlapping cultural contexts that influence clients' beliefs, values, behaviors, and motivations within a historical and sociopolitical context, even when clients themselves may not be fully aware of these influences.

In this therapeutic context, liberation-based healing empowers individuals to traverse bridges toward empowerment (DeGruy, 2005). Connections that intricately weave together within each woman's internal landscape allow for an exploration of past traumas and present dynamics, and link the women together externally, forming new relationships and shared understanding. Black women, bound by a common racial identity, use these bridges to explore shared experiences of oppression while recognizing their unique challenges. The concept of intergenerational trauma underlies these bridges, offering insight into how historical injustices have impacted each woman and her community (DeGruy, 2005). These bridges enable a comprehensive exploration of intergenerational trauma, allowing Black women to navigate their shared history toward healing and resilience (Crenshaw, 1989; DeGruy, 2005).

Communal healing, a key element of intersectionality, acknowledges the interconnected nature of individuals' identities and their communities. It emphasizes that healing is a collective journey, recognizing shared experiences of pain and joy within communities with shared identities. Incorporating communal healing circles and groups into service offerings and marketing efforts allows art therapist entrepreneurs to demonstrate their commitment to intersectionality and social justice. Communal groups, led by art therapists, serve as powerful tools for promoting their practice, embodying intersectional principles, and fostering liberation-based healing. These offerings show the art therapist's expertise in creating inclusive, intersectional spaces, positioning them as community advocates and partners who understand the importance of addressing diverse identities.

## TAILORING SERVICES FROM AN INTERSECTIONAL APPROACH

I have found that intersectional marketing is not just a tool for outreach, but that intersectionality is a philosophy that extends into the core of my practice, influencing every aspect from community engagement to clinical services. A prime example of this is the communal healing group I previously mentioned, which served as an intersectional marketing initiative through community outreach. It was within this group that I first met the client I'll refer to as "Dorothy."

From 2018 to 2020, the country reeled under a number of high-profile police killings of Black people. These events deeply affected Dorothy. The targeted outreach I initiated, which highlighted the inclusivity and cultural sensitivity of my practice, resonated with Dorothy's needs and ultimately allowed her to find a safe space to process her trauma. She indicated she was drawn to my practice because of the emphasis on addressing the unique challenges faced by marginalized communities. In this section, I will discuss how my marketing efforts, rooted in the principles of intersectionality, assured clients that my practice is a space where their experiences will be understood, and identities respected.

As an art therapist and practice owner, I am committed to ensuring that the themes of intersectionality and inclusivity are reflected in all aspects of my business and across the services I provide. I use client-centered approaches, which prioritize clients' needs, and focus on empathy, active listening, and unconditional positive regard. This method provides a secure space for clients to explore their thoughts, emotions, and identities, especially when considering intersectionality (Davis, 2008; Sue & Sue, 2016). Through this commitment, I seamlessly integrate intersectionality from my marketing to the services I provide, ensuring every client feels understood and supported.

As we explored Dorothy's complex identities, we delved into her relationship with the Christian upbringing that had shaped her. Her connection with Christianity revealed a complex narrative intertwined with the historical legacy of slavery and systemic racism (Williams et al., 2019). Dorothy also shared that the emphasis on a "white, male God" within

Christianity challenged her ability to fully embrace her femininity within the faith, perpetuating a patriarchal, Eurocentric worldview that marginalized her identity as a spiritual and Black woman. However, within Christianity, Dorothy found empowerment, hope, and solace, and she acknowledged its role in inspiring the civil rights movement. She grappled with embracing a faith historically used to legitimize her oppression while striving to reinterpret it to reflect her experiences, identities, and aspirations for a more inclusive and just world.

During our sessions, I encouraged Dorothy to seek spiritual role models, individuals, images, or concepts that resonated with her unique intersectionality. Her exploration led her to the intriguing feminine-based spirituality of the Black Madonna, a title referring to sacred icons or statues of the Virgin Mary often depicted with dark or black skin (Birnbaum, 2002). These revered images hold significant religious and cultural significance across various regions of Europe. Notable examples include the Black Madonna of Częstochowa in Poland, Our Lady of Montserrat in Spain, and the Black Madonna of Chartres in France (Birnbaum, 2002).

The origin and meaning of the Black Madonna continue to be the subject of debate among scholars and theologians. The dark skin of these statues is often interpreted symbolically, representing a connection to the Earth, fertility, and the mystery of creation (Birnbaum, 2002). Some scholars attribute the black color to centuries of candle soot accumulation or specific materials used in their creation (Birnbaum, 2002). Others view them as symbols of multiculturalism and religious syncretism, while some emphasize their religious importance.

The Black Madonna's dark skin can serve as a symbol of racial identity. For Dorothy, creating a visual and spiritual representation of her Blackness through artistic expression provided a sense of belonging, pride, and an exploration and celebration of her intersectional identities, particularly through her interpretation of the Black Madonna (Figure 5.2). The Black Madonna's dark skin can serve as a symbol of racial identity. Figure 5.2, created by Dorothy, embodies her ideal spiritual entity, providing a powerful platform for her to explore and challenge traditional gender norms and roles. The Black Madonna, as a representation of the divine feminine, offered a space for discussion of the intersection of gender and spirituality within a Black context.

In my role as an art therapist, I recognized the transformative potential of Dorothy's artwork featuring the Black Madonna. Like a bridge, it connected us to discussions about her racial identity, experiences of racism, and their profound impact on her mental well-being. Through this creative process, she embarked on a spiritual journey, addressing her questions and inner struggles. Art therapists, guided by principles of respect and cultural humility (Paine et al., 2018), can assist clients in uncovering meaning, finding inner peace, and gaining a deeper understanding of their spirituality.

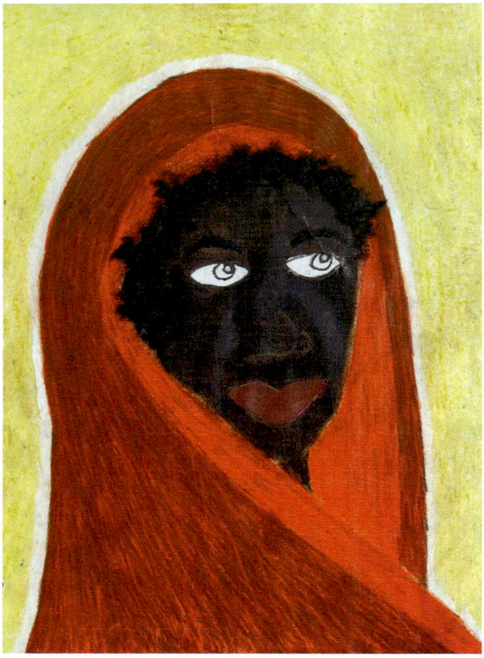

***Figure 5.2*** *Black Madonna.*
*Note:* Dorothy's artwork, depicting the Black Madonna with interactive, tactile hair.

By creating a safe and nonthreatening environment, I allowed Dorothy to explore deeply personal and sometimes challenging subjects. This approach enabled her to fully express the rich tapestry of identities within this inclusive space. She articulated her vision for the Black Madonna's skin as "dark and rich," akin to fertile soil, achieved by blending brown and black colored pencils. This choice was central, as it allowed her to convey her personal interpretation.

Dorothy exhibited a particular fascination with rendering the Black Madonna's hair in a way that reflected her perception of an African woman. To achieve this, she used black yarn, cut into small pieces, and skillfully glued to the paper. Furthermore, she aimed to capture "feminine beauty" within this divine figure. This intention manifested in the rendering of full mauve-colored lips and eyes adorned with crescent moon shapes, their gaze soft and distant, extending beyond the viewer's perspective. To complete her depiction, Dorothy fashioned a wrap or scarf that covered the top of the Black Madonna's head, gently grazing her chin before vanishing off the page. The color of this wrap was a nuanced shade of red, meticulously rendered with black pencil strokes, imparting a tactile texture reminiscent of rough cloth.

Overall, the imagery of the Black Madonna served as a profound and multifaceted bridge for Dorothy's introspective journey into her Black identity, gender experiences, and spirituality, all viewed through the illuminating lens of intersectionality. A transformative process for a deeper comprehension of the intricate layers of her identity but also a catalyst for healing, empowerment, and self-acceptance. The Black Madonna, with her diverse symbolism and cultural significance, proved to be a powerful muse for Dorothy's self-discovery, ultimately guiding her toward a place of greater understanding and resilience.

## CONCLUSION

In conclusion, the profound benefits of intersectionality in our art therapy endeavors extend far beyond the therapeutic process itself. By embracing an intersectional lens, we can create more accessible and inclusive marketing strategies that resonate with diverse audiences. This approach not only attracts a wider range of clients but also strengthens our reputation as culturally responsive and compassionate practitioners. Much like the various components of a bridge working in harmony to create a stronger and more resilient structure, recognizing the different identities within intersectionality fortifies our practice.

Implementing intersectionality in the marketing of my private practice has significantly exceeded my expectations for referrals. By showcasing a commitment to inclusive and intersectional approaches, I have attracted a diverse clientele seeking an affirming therapeutic space. This success has allowed me to expand my practice by adding clinicians who align with these principles. In addition, I use intersectional concepts in the supervision I give to art therapists, which has fostered a supportive environment that recognizes the complexities of the therapists' identities. This approach not only enhances the quality of services but also strengthens the sense of community within my practice. Looking forward, I envision leveraging intersectionality to further expand my business practices and social justice entrepreneurship ideas, including developing innovative programs, partnerships, and initiatives that address diverse needs, promote inclusivity, and contribute to positive social change.

Through this unity of differences, we can promote and market our art therapy endeavors as nurturing environments where healing and self-expression flourish, ultimately making our programs or practices a beacon of holistic and transformative therapy. Each aspect of identity serves as a crucial support, reinforcing our commitment to inclusivity and understanding. Together, they build a bridge to healing and self-discovery that is not only sturdy but also beautiful in its diversity and resilience.

## REFERENCES

Almeida, R. V., & Tubbs, C. Y. (2020). Intersectionality: A liberation-based healing perspective. In K. S. Wampler, R. B. Miller, & R. B. Seedall (Eds.), *The handbook of systemic family therapy: Volume 1* (pp. 227–250). Wiley.

American Psychological Association. (2017). *Multicultural guidelines: An ecological approach to context, identity, and intersectionality.* Retrieved from www.apa.org/about/policy/multicultural-guidelines.pdf

American Psychological Association. (2023). *Equity, diversity, and inclusion: Inclusive language guide* (2nd ed.). Retrieved from www.apa.org/about/apa/equity-diversity-inclusion/language-guide.pdf

Art Therapy Credentials Board. (2021). *Code of ethics, conduct, and disciplinary procedures.* Retrieved from https://atcb.org/wp-content/uploads/2023/12/ATCB-Code-of-Ethics-Conduct-DisciplinaryProcedures-fixed.pdf

Birnbaum, L. (2002). *Dark mother: African origins and godmothers.* iUniverse.

Collins, P. H., & Bilge, S. (2016). *Intersectionality.* Polity Press.

Cook, B. L., McGuire, T., & Miranda, J. (2007). Measuring trends in mental health care disparities, 2000–2004. *58*(12), 1521–1632. Retrieved from https://psychiatryonline.org/doi/full/10.1176/ps.2007.58.12.1533

Crenshaw, K. (1989). Demarginalizing the intersection of race and sex: A black feminist critique of antidiscrimination doctrine, feminist theory, and antiracist politics. *University of Chicago Legal Forum, 1989*(1), 139–167.

Crenshaw, K. (1991). Mapping the margins: Intersectionality, identity politics, and violence against women of color. *Stanford Law Review, 43*(6), 1241–1299.

Datlen, G. W., & Pandolfi, C. (2020). Developing an online art therapy group for learning disabled young adults using WhatsApp. *International Journal of Art Therapy, 25*(4), 192–201.

Davis, K. (2008). Intersectionality as buzzword: A sociology of science perspective on what makes a feminist theory successful. *Feminist Theory, 9*(1), 67–85.

DeGruy, J. (2005). *Post traumatic slave syndrome: America's legacy of enduring injury and healing.* Uptone Press.

Eastwood, C., McDonald, A., Turner, D., & Vernon, P. (2023). Intersectionality and art therapy. *International Journal of Art Therapy, 28*(1–2), 2–6. https://doi.org/10.1080/17454832.2023.2221517

Ginwright, S. (2018). *The future of healing: Shifting from trauma informed care to healing centered engagement.* Medium. Retrieved from https://ginwright.medium.com/the-future-of-healing-shifting-from-trauma-informed-care-to-healing-centered-engagement-634f557ce69c

Gipson, L. R. (2015). Is cultural competence enough? Deepening social justice pedagogy in art therapy. *Art Therapy: Journal of the American Art Therapy, 32*(3), 143–145.

Imran, A. (2022). Why addressing digital inequality should be a priority. *The Electronic Journal of Information Systems in Developing Countries, 89*(3), 1–12. Retrieved from https://onlinelibrary.wiley.com/doi/full/10.1002/isd2.12255

Karcher, O. P. (2017). Sociopolitical oppression, trauma, and healing: Moving toward a social justice art therapy framework. *Art Therapy: Journal of the American Art Therapy Association, 34*(3), 123–128.

Malchiodi, C. A. (2018). *The handbook of art therapy and digital technology*. Jessica Kingsley.

Paine, D. R., Moon, S. H., Hauge, D. J., & Sandage, S. J. (2018). Cultural and racial perspectives on positive psychologies of humility. In N. J. L. Brown, T. Lomas, & F. J. Eiroa-Orosa (Eds.), *The Routledge international handbook of critical positive psychology* (pp. 281–298). Routledge.

Practice Solutions. (2016). *Sliding scale fees: Implementing income based pricing*. Practice Solutions. Retrieved from www.practicesol.com/single-post/sliding-scale-fees-implementing-income-based-pricing

Roger, C. R. (1957). The necessary and sufficient conditions of therapeutic personality change. *Journal of Consulting Psychology, 21*(2), 95–103.

Rushin, K. (2015). The bridge poem. In C. Moraga & G. E. Anzaldúa (Eds.), *This bridge called my back: Writing by radical women of color* (4th ed., pp. xxxiii–xxxiv). SUNY Press.

Shafir, T., Orkibi, H., Baker, F. A., Gussak, D., & Kaimal, G. (2020). Editorial: The state of the art in creative arts therapies. *Frontiers in Psychology, 11*(68), 1–4. Retrieved from www.frontiersin.org/journals/psychology/articles/10.3389/fpsyg.2020.00068/full

Sue, D. W., & Sue, D. (2016). *Counseling the culturally diverse: Theory and practice* (7th ed.). Wiley.

Talwar, S. (2010). An intersectional framework for race, class, gender and culture in art therapy. *Art Therapy: Journal of the American Art Therapy Association, 27*(1), 11–17.

Talwar, S., & Sajnani, N. (2022). Intersectionality and the ethics of care in the creative arts therapies. *Arts in Psychotherapy, 80*, 10194.

Tomlinson, B. (2013). To tell the truth and not get trapped: Desire, distance, and intersectionality at the scene of argument. *Signs: Journal of Women in Culture and Society, 38*(4), 993–1017.

Williams, M. T., Rosen, D. C., & Kanter, J. W. (2019). *Eliminating race-based mental health disparities*. Context Press.

Wilson, L., Riley, S., & Wadeson, H. (1984). Art therapy supervision. *Art Therapy, 1*(3), 100–105. Retrieved from www.tandfonline.com/doi/abs/10.1080/07421656.1984.10758761

Wright, T., & Wright, K. (2017). Exploring the benefits of intersectional feminist social justice approaches in art psychotherapy. *Arts in Psychotherapy, 54*(2017), 7–14.

Zappa, A. (2017). Beyond erasure: The ethics of art therapy research with trans and gender-independent people. *Art Therapy: Journal of the American Art Therapy Association, 34*(3), 129–134.

*Chapter* **6**

# Creating a Self-Contained Mobile Art Therapy Facility

*Lisa Lounsbury*

## INCUBATION

My name is Lisa Lounsbury, and I am the founder and executive director of Art Lab Rx, LLC, a mental health agency founded in 2015 with a focus on delivering art therapy services within the state of Minnesota. I am a licensed marriage and family therapist and a board-certified art therapist. I received my master's degree in 2014 from Adler Graduate School in Minnetonka, MN.

It took a village to create my business and many people played a part, as did my faith. I took many pathways earlier in my career and I will share some of these experiences to provide context for the variety of skills I learned. Before Art Lab Rx and Maggie (my mobile art therapy bus), I held many jobs and had a range of professional experiences, all of which gave me invaluable skills. During high school, I studied in Guatemala for six months, where I learned to speak Spanish and developed a new worldview. As an executive secretary for a local newspaper, I learned business communication protocols and managerial skills. When I co-owned a cooperative gallery, I learned to negotiate rent and space with the building owners and administered oversight of the artist-members affiliated with the shared studio, gallery, and retail spaces. For a few years, I managed painting teams around the country for a scenic painting studio. Through these experiences, I learned about managing big projects alongside other tradespeople with shared goals, and how to tightly pack a road box with all the necessary materials and tools for an on-site painting gig. I also volunteered at a local puppet theater where I learned to create small-scale puppet shows that would be tucked inside suitcases, which would shift and transform into life-size shows and large-scale puppets supported by

DOI: 10.4324/9781032615776-7

backpack structures. I learned a tremendous amount about how to create something out of nothing, and that work proved helpful when my church asked me to design and facilitate a puppet ministry program for a mission trip. These roles and experiences trained me to be flexible, innovative, use space to its maximum, and be involved in the community.

I experienced some hardship after being let go from a stable job that had supported me and my son when I was a newly divorced single mom. Shortly after losing my job, and before becoming an art therapist, I facilitated an art workshop for a local addiction treatment center. The response from the women in the group helped me realize the tremendous impact the process of art making has on a person's self-awareness. I knew this was juicy, and I also knew I needed to get an education to support what I thought this was—art therapy. I had no job and no college education. I believe God provided the way, because I was blessed to earn scholarships and grants that helped me to attend college.

The gestational period of my business journey started with my entry into formal education in my mid-forties. I began working toward my Associate of Arts Degree in the fall of 2008, and I completed my graduate program from Adler Graduate School, in marriage and family therapy with an emphasis in art therapy, in March 2014.

While in school, I continued facilitating healing arts groups to the same local addiction treatment center. Other addiction recovery programs heard about my services and hired me. My contracting client base grew and I negotiated to get those jobs approved as internship sites when applicable.

## INFANCY

While providing art therapy services inside addiction treatment facilities, it became clear that there was a need for something different. The spaces available to me were usually inadequate, and I was often working in cramped rooms dedicated to other purposes. Clients would often leave paintbrushes and cups in the bathroom and would not return to the group. The rooms were usually not private, and staff would come in and out. If we did have use of a larger conference room, we had more table space for clients to make art, but these rooms were also not private, were usually carpeted (inevitably someone would spill paint and cause a stain) and had no sink. Some agencies provided us space in a larger social room, separating us by only an office divider wall; this situation usually became very loud. Clients were frustrated, especially if they were in the middle of sharing about an emotional experience, and managing the ethics of privacy during these sessions was impossible.

It was very difficult to find a space in any contracting agency that was adequate for art therapy. It was a physical effort to bring in all the art materials and tools for each week's sessions and a struggle to maintain a consistent ambience for the experience.

Lisa Hinz (2009) talks about how some hesitant participants will comment that art making is difficult, "For most individuals, being asked to use art media, perhaps for the first time in many years, brings up overwhelming feelings of uncertainty and insecurity. Claiming lack of artistic ability may be the only way clients think they can control these uncomfortable emotions" (p. 233). These are real and powerful anxieties about beginning an art therapy session. Being in a physically comfortable, contained setting where clients have easy access to materials allows clients to feel a sense of mastery over their creative space.

To counter the unpredictable nature of the settings where I was providing services, I applied thought and care to how I created a safe space for clients. During each session, I would place the art materials and tools in the exact same place. The consistency of the set-up promoted a sense of security and reliability, helping to build trust in the therapeutic relationship and process. Each session would begin with a grounding exercise, followed by a description of the topic of the day and a short description or reading from relevant materials. Clients would have time to use the materials provided to create art and I would provide nature sounds for ambience. When art-making time was over, I would invite clients to do a "gallery walk" where they would walk clockwise around the tables to view each other's work. Clients who were willing would be invited to share their experiences, we would have a discussion, and close with another grounding exercise. This method, which helped to promote a sense of trust, has become "the Art Lab way."

## VISION AND INNOVATION

One afternoon, I drove past a building that I thought would make a great healing arts center. I began to pray but stopped and asked myself, "What if I'm wrong?" Moments later, I heard a small voice whisper, "Put it on a bus." Excited, thinking this was a divine message, I said, "That's brilliant, a bus could solve all my problems." Thus, the messy childhood stage began.

The vision for my project was to create a completely self-contained mobile art therapy facility where clients would have everything they needed for the session. I was finishing my master's degree. I needed a lot of help, a good plan, and money. I enrolled in a business plan writing course offered by a local nonprofit agency called Women Venture (WV), which was specifically for women starting businesses. I learned about many areas of owning a business including types of entities, market analysis, assessing feasibility, business accounting, advertising, marketing, regulations and licensing, finances, specifics of my industry, and differences between for-profit and nonprofit businesses. Taking the business plan course provided me with a more well-rounded picture of entrepreneurship in general, and it specifically helped me identify areas where I needed to do more research.

As part of the WV course, I needed to register my business. I completed a name search on the Minnesota Secretary of State's website to make sure Art Lab Rx was available, and I filed the assumed name paperwork with the state of Minnesota. As part of the approval process, I was required to publish a notice in a legal newspaper, one authorized to publish public notices and legal advertisements, for two consecutive days, after which they gave me an affidavit of publication, and my business name was official. I chose to become an LLC instead of a nonprofit because I did not want to have a board of directors, and my research indicated I would not be able to facilitate the programming if I served on the board.

Having a financial plan was one of the most important parts of the business plan. It took effort to plan for each step that was needed to retrofit the bus. Budgeting for what I wanted on the bus was one thing. I discovered what was actually needed for the bus after I bought one. My original retrofit plan was based on an estimate provided by someone who did retrofitting for a living. He was a referral who turned out to be not trustworthy, and I lost $500 as well as some forward movement.

The rest of the professionals I worked with were trustworthy and respectful of me as a business owner with a big idea. I was referred to a reputable bus dealer, JD, who spent time talking with me and asking questions about my plan. Some of his questions helped me establish my plan more firmly, and his questions became a type of coaching. He helped me understand which line of buses would fit my needs and would also have parts available for easy and less expensive repair.

## ADOLESCENCE

In order to build capital to buy a bus, I needed to continue working with treatment centers and save my income. Business grew as I added additional treatment centers, and I hired two interns to facilitate groups. In December 2017, I was able to purchase a 2000 MCI 102DL3D coach bus with a newly rebuilt engine. The bus is 45 feet long and 11½ feet tall, with a wheelchair lift and a bathroom in the back. I named the bus Maggie after Margaret Naumburg, one of the early leaders in the art therapy field.

Our WV cohort networked well and helped to refer other helpful professionals. Through this network, I established connections to an art director,

Susan Ebertowski, a woodworker artist, David Aichinger, and received a referral to a local bank, BankCherokee, which catered to women-owned businesses. I brought my business plan to that bank and asked for a Small Business Association loan to retrofit the bus, using the bus itself as collateral. I also received a small loan from WV. This funding provided most of the money to retrofit the bus. Because business overhead was low, and I was blessed to rely on my husband's income for our living expenses, I was able to continue investing in Art Lab Rx.

Maggie needed a complete transformation on the inside and out. Family and friends helped with some demolition of the interior, but I had not thought about what I would do with the salvaged seats and overhead bins. Thankfully, JD kept everything as a trade for the cost of labor to remove them. Once the seats were gone—except for two seats to the right of the driver, for any passengers who might ride along, and to allow for a type of "waiting room"—the carpet was removed. We covered the ceiling with a white metal sheeting and painted the side walls white. The entire inside became a blank canvas. The interior seemed huge, and it was easy to see my vision of clients working on a variety of creative projects in the space.

Unplanned expenses were bound to occur and, thankfully, I allocated funds to this area in the business plan. Insurance was one; it was necessary and more expensive than expected. I found an agency that would provide comprehensive and collision insurance for the bus itself, along with general liability for any accidents when participants were in the bus. This expense was in addition to my professional liability insurance. Another unplanned expense was the floor of the bus. It was in decent shape except for the long metal channels that secured the seats in place. Those channels would be troublesome if we wanted to roll anything on the floor, so we decided to cover the whole floor with plywood, which is fairly inexpensive, easy to cut, install, and seal. Each unplanned expense was worth the investment and my vision of the finished bus became more focused.

In consideration of the bus interior, the group art therapy session space, I initially wanted an art table in the middle with chairs around it so participants could face each other. Each time we tried to configure a working scenario, space became a problem. The arched ceiling design did not allow enough headspace for people to walk around the table while others were seated. It was frustrating, but after we let go of the center table idea, we focused on a desk with locking casters that would provide the art material storage containment I was looking for and the mobility of configuring the desks around the interior space.

There were several aspects to consider when designing the desks including which art materials, tools, and equipment I wanted the clients to have at hand, size requirements for the desks to fit on the lift, and what the work surface dimensions would be to give the clients the best experience possible. After choosing my materials and tools, I gave them to David Aichinger, and he began designing. After nine months and several iterations and adorable small-scale models, we developed a customized design that would fulfill the functional needs of the space. The desks provide plenty of work surface which can be converted from a horizontal surface to an easel by lifting the center section. A wide center drawer stores sheets of paper and flat nesting trays which hold watercolors, chalk, and oil pastels. There is also a pull-out shelf for additional work surface while using the easel feature. Three drawers on either side hold small blow dryers, custom-made hot glue caddies, acrylic paint, and more. Other custom-made caddies hold markers, colored pencils, paint brushes, and a cup for water. The desks are secured to a side ledge of the bus interior with special cam-locks that are easily adjusted to unlock and move the desks. Self-locking marine hardware was installed on all drawers and cabinet doors to keep them closed while traveling. After using these desks for several years, there is very little I would change. The desks are a work of art on their own.

I chose a bus that came with a wheelchair lift and was interested in what we could do to make our space both user-friendly and compliant with the Americans with Disabilities Act. I connected with the Great Lakes ADA Center to learn what it would take to make that possible. Although ADA requirements stated that only one desk needed to be wheelchair accessible, all desks were designed with the necessary leg height, chair width, and open foot space desktop to accommodate a wheelchair. The desks were also mounted on locking casters, so they could be reconfigured with all the desks on one side, allowing individuals to get on the bus through the lift and maneuver to select a desk. Benck Mechanical expanded the bathroom space to accommodate most wheelchairs and raised the height of the toilet seat by three inches. Aichinger built a beautiful, large door for the newly enlarged bathroom area. Benck also installed a sink with fresh and grey water tanks, a generator to handle all of the electrical needs, and a heating and air conditioning unit (HVAC) for us to provide services year-round.

Several other small amenities were added to make the space fully functional with the desired ambience for a session. We completed the interior by installing epoxy flooring with plastic confetti pieces that match the colorful graphics on the exterior of the bus. The floor is colorful, nonslip, and helps to hide any paint spills. The interior has a clean, inviting feel that I describe as a Scandinavian industrial look, as seen in Figure 6.1.

Getting the proper license plate was tricky. I had several conversations with a number of supervisors at the Department of Motor Vehicles about how to classify the bus now that it was no longer a passenger vehicle. During that discussion, I had to decide between registering as an interstate

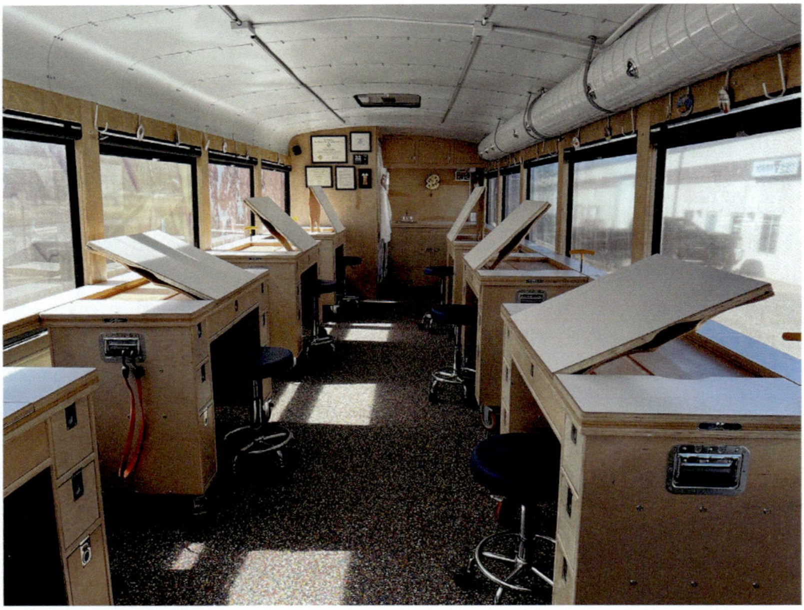

***Figure 6.1*** *Maggie's Interior.*

*Note*: Interior view of Maggie with its inviting, clean, Scandinavian industrial look. This shows the versatility of the desktops, the nonslip epoxy floor, and the white HVAC tubing; in the back, there is the lighted sink area with its storage above.

vehicle—which would include a more expensive license plate and require tracking and reporting miles to other states—or an intrastate vehicle with no tracking, no reporting, and a less expensive plate. I concluded that there would be enough work for us within our state.

The exterior of the bus was very important since it would be my company's billboard. The graphic designer, Susan Ebertowski, whom I hired from our WV cohort, provided art direction for Art Lab's website, marketing collateral package, and the idea for the bus wrap. She had connections to a photographer who shot my original artwork at a high resolution. JD provided a referral to Creative Color, an agency that does large print vehicle wraps. They printed the image onto adhesive vinyl for the colorful, eye-catching wrap on the outside of Maggie, including perforated sections for the windows to promote privacy. The perforations meant people could not see into the bus, but participants could still look out. The wrap did require Maggie's exterior surface to be smoothed out before it could be applied, which was another unanticipated expense, but well worth it. The exterior of Maggie now is colorful and inviting, as can be seen from Figure 6.2.

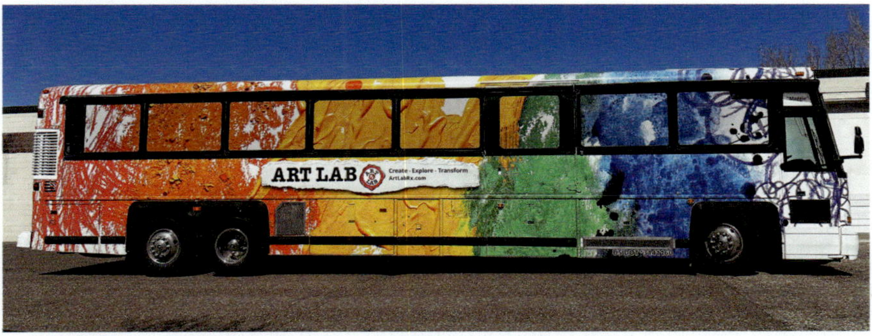


***Figure 6.2*** *Maggie's Exterior.*

*Note:* Side view of Maggie with her colorful, inviting vinyl wrap installed by Creative Color, using original artwork created by Lisa Lounsbury.

## ART THERAPY ON A BUS

When on Maggie, clients experience a private therapy setting that is also a self-contained art studio. By putting the studio on a bus, I am able to work with clients who need me to go to them. A mobile facility breaks down the barriers of transportation and accessibility that may hinder some people from participating in therapy. A mobile facility also expands the offerings of partnering agencies who can now provide art therapy services without having to create their own studio space in-house. When contracting with an agency to provide services on Maggie, I needed to ensure they have a level area where Maggie can be parked. If the bus is to be on a city street, permits and adequate parking for the 45-foot vehicle must be secured prior to our arrival.

During a typical group session on the bus, clients enter and get settled by hanging their coats and putting on an apron. I give an orientation to the space, the desks, the HVAC system, and their supplies. We engage in a mindfulness breathing exercise and I describe the focus topic for the session. Clients then start making art. Clients are free to move around the bus to use the bathroom, get additional materials that may be laid out on the back counter, and use the sink. Clients also can hang their two-dimensional art above their desks to view. Clients move their stools back to create a type of semi-circle to see each other during group discussion about the artwork. Wood (2000) said, "Being set apart from the everyday provides the physical space needed for mental reflection" (p. 40). He added that, "The life difficulties experienced by many clients are extreme, yet the availability of a studio can add to their capacity to face what they feel. This is because the actual making of art can engender a sense of thoughtful absorption and this can make it possible to reflect upon what is felt and then possibly even see the feelings in the artwork" (p. 43). Having a controlled environment in a contained art studio space assists with thoughtful absorption.

## MANAGING RISK

There were several risks to creating a mobile art facility. There were knowledge gaps that required me to be comfortable with uncertainty, relying on flexibility, developing entrepreneurial skills in real-time, local competition, Minnesota weather, and following my faith in the vision.

One risk of a new business is that you may have competition in the same space. I did research to identify if there were other mobile art therapy services that would serve as competition to Art Lab Rx. I found two other mobile art businesses. Wayne Ramirez (1989) created a mobile arts bus in the Virgin Islands during the 1970s. His arts bus featured musicians, visual artists, art therapists, and special education teachers working together to serve the community's children. This was not a risk; the success of his project and personal conversations with him served as a source of encouragement. I also found a local business on a bus that focused on providing after-school art-making opportunities for children who lived in housing projects. This business was not providing art therapy services and was specifically focused on working with children, thus not determined to not be in direct competition with Art Lab Rx.

The Minnesota winters can be severe and hard on a bus. I needed to find permanent parking, specifically temperature-controlled parking, for the winter. At the time I launched Maggie, Adler Graduate School allowed me to park Maggie in their lot during the summer and I provided learning opportunities for students who served as interns with Art Lab Rx. I also provided tours and talks during events at the school.

Perhaps one of the biggest risks was to follow my faith, knowing that this was a call from God to "put it on a bus" without having community partners to join with me yet. Being such a unique opportunity, it did not take long to gain partnerships in both rural areas of Minnesota and the inner city.

Having the mindset of an artist and a businesswoman allowed me to move fluidly through times where expectations shifted, and regulations required something unexpected. Flexibility was an important business skill to have while developing the mobile art therapy facility because I was making decisions while I was learning. Effectively communicating my vision to others was sometimes a challenge, but the more I trusted their expertise, the better our collaborations went.

The experience of creating a mobile facility was enhanced by my mentors and the community of people who provided their support, skill, and expertise to bring it to life. Those connections contributed to the further growth of Art Lab Rx. I continue to provide internship opportunities for students at Adler Graduate School and have expanded this to include students from other art therapy programs. I have also provided mentorship and guidance to several individuals who desire to start their own mobile service. It is my hope that this helps to expand mobile art therapy services into other communities.

## TEEN YEARS

Art Lab Rx launched in July 2015, and because of our partnerships with local agencies striving to fulfill needs they see in the community, we have been able to grow and serve more people every year. Art Lab Rx has served the mental health needs of thousands by our partnerships with local addiction treatment centers, government offices, schools, and other mental health organizations both through in-house delivery and on Maggie. I have weekly sessions at contracting entities and full-day events where the clients participate on the bus for an hour at a time, or fluidly throughout the day for an open studio wellness day. Art Lab Rx crafts programming that works best for the organization and their population.

The 2022 American Art Therapy Association (AATA) national conference was held in Minneapolis, MN. I parked Maggie next to the hotel, which increased visibility and awareness of our programs. My interns and I gave tours during the event for participants from around the country. Through this networking initiative, we developed a new partnership with Premier Arts Collective (PAC), a faith-based nonprofit that supports programming in South Carolina, Minneapolis, and other parts of the world. As a result of our participation in the conference and networking, we began a new partnership with PAC in 2023. PAC provides financial support that enables us to bring art therapy to more people and agencies in Minnesota who otherwise might not have been able to afford it.

Maggie is a moving billboard and causes excitement and interest wherever she goes. There have been many opportunities for us to assist with fundraising efforts for some of our partners by bringing Maggie and providing tours with opportunities to make small artworks that are made into lapel pins. We support our partner's cause while also raising awareness of art therapy. Our participation in outreach activities and events also promotes visibility for our business and helps us to establish new connections and partnerships.

## CONCLUSION

In the ten years Art Lab Rx has been operating, we have reached adulthood. Art Lab Rx employs a team of a dozen professionals doing wonderful transformative work. We have addressed the mental health needs of our community through art therapy services in-house at several partnering agencies as well as by bringing Maggie to places surrounding Minneapolis. Now Maggie has a permanent temperature-controlled parking space in our converted machine shop warehouse, and people can come to us for art therapy services. This space includes a front gallery waiting area, an office, two bathrooms, and a huge group studio space where we provide a variety of art therapy groups and wellness workshops on-site. Our partnerships are increasing, and along with this growth, we are able to provide more internship opportunities for art therapy graduate students.

Maggie herself has at least another ten years of operation, if not more, with good maintenance. In the future, we hope to find a physical space where we can create several private therapy offices, an open studio group space, a small retail space with coffee service, a large garage for Maggie, a garden for a walking labyrinth, and nature-based therapy. This could become a collective of art therapists and wellness professionals working toward the same goal of overall wellness. I envision hiring someone to manage the business while I shift to more of a supervisor/mentor role and continue providing opportunities for other professionals and students. I also dream of creating a franchise for many more Maggie's around the world.

As a community of professionals, we transformed Maggie from a touring coach bus into a traveling art therapy clinic, and now, a greasy machine shop into a fun art therapy space. We now can fulfill the saying, "We go to you, or you come to us!"

## REFERENCES

Hinz, L. D. (2009). *Expressive therapies continuum: A framework for using art in therapy*. Routledge.

Ramirez, W. (1989). *The little island school bus that became the "arts mobile"*. Self-Published.

Wood, C. (2000). The significance of studios. *International Journal of Art Therapy: Inscape*, *5*(2), 40–53. https://doi.org/10.1080/17454830008413089

Chapter 7

# Queer Coalition Building in the Creative Arts Therapies

## A Personal Reflection and Introduction

*Zachary D. Van Den Berg*

As both artists and therapists, art therapists are uniquely positioned to respond to the needs of our communities by collaborating across differences to craft systemic interventions that resonate deeply, ensuring equitable and ethical access to care (Talwar, 2015). This work of social entrepreneurship (Newey, 2017) spans the initiation, provision, and maintenance of varied art therapy services (DeLucia et al., 2020, 2021). Yet, absent critical self-reflexivity and humility, even the most well-intentioned care initiatives risk perpetuating systems of marginalization and harm (Hetherington, 2020). A radical approach to social entrepreneurship, therefore, does not merely produce health services in communities but critically intertwines care indelibly with transformative justice, challenging us to examine the dynamic social terrains we navigate both personally and professionally (Van Den Berg & Anderson, 2023).

For queer-identified art therapists, especially those working within their lesbian, gay, bisexual, transgender, queer, questioning, intersex, asexual, plus (LGBTQIA+) communities, there exists a profound connection to the lived experiences of gender and sexual diversity—a parallel to the lives of our clients that is frequently overlooked in traditional professional and training contexts (Van Den Berg, 2023). Guided by these shared experiences, LGBTQIA+-identified art therapists have often been compelled to envision and implement alternative theoretical, ethical, and practical approaches to affirm these unique cultural considerations (Anderson, 2020). Despite their significance, these contributions frequently go unrecognized, a form of erasure that not only underscores the challenges posed by dominant cis-heteronormative narratives within professional discourse but also reflects broader sociocultural, historical, and political paradigms

DOI: 10.4324/9781032615776-8

(Van Den Berg, 2024; Zappa, 2017). Addressing these issues across the scholarship and organizational spheres of our profession is crucial.

## OVERVIEW

This chapter begins with a reflection on my journey of establishing the Coalition for Queer Creative Arts Therapies—an online forum that has since flourished into an independent nonprofit organization and a digital professional development resource, distinct from its origins on social media platforms. I will then chart the evolution of Expressing Pride (our annual symposium) from a fledgling idea to an annual, free, virtual event that champions queer-affirming practices within the arts therapies community.

The experiences I will share with you are driven by a profound commitment to creating spaces where voices at the margins can find resonance, affirmation, and empowerment as well as examples of how social entrepreneurship can drive the queer creative arts therapies movement forward. They illustrate an important interplay of necessity and vision—a vision that seeks not only to challenge existing paradigms but also to offer an alternative; a realm of coalition-building and queer kinship across the creative arts therapies. Reflecting upon these insights necessitates acknowledging my positionality: I am white, late-20s, Jewish, queer, genderqueer, neurodivergent, and nondisabled, and I was born a U.S. citizen, raised in a middle-class, cis-heteronormative suburb of Austin, Texas.

## PAINTING QUEER FAMILY PORTRAITS

In my undergraduate studies, I began to embrace queerness as both an identity and an epistemological stance, finding in queer theory and history the language to shape previously ineffable desires and experiences. I embarked on a deeply personal project: the creation of a portrait series featuring queer families, which served as a medium for critiquing and reimagining the constructs of family within a queer context. One of these portraits captures my partner, our two dogs, and me (Figure 7.1).

This endeavor coincided with my enrollment in undergraduate art therapy courses, which deepened my already introspective art-making practice. These courses offered a structured framework that enhanced my understanding and articulation of personal and collective queer narratives through art, highlighting the role of self-portraiture in my journey as an act of resistance and place-making within a cis-heterosexist society.

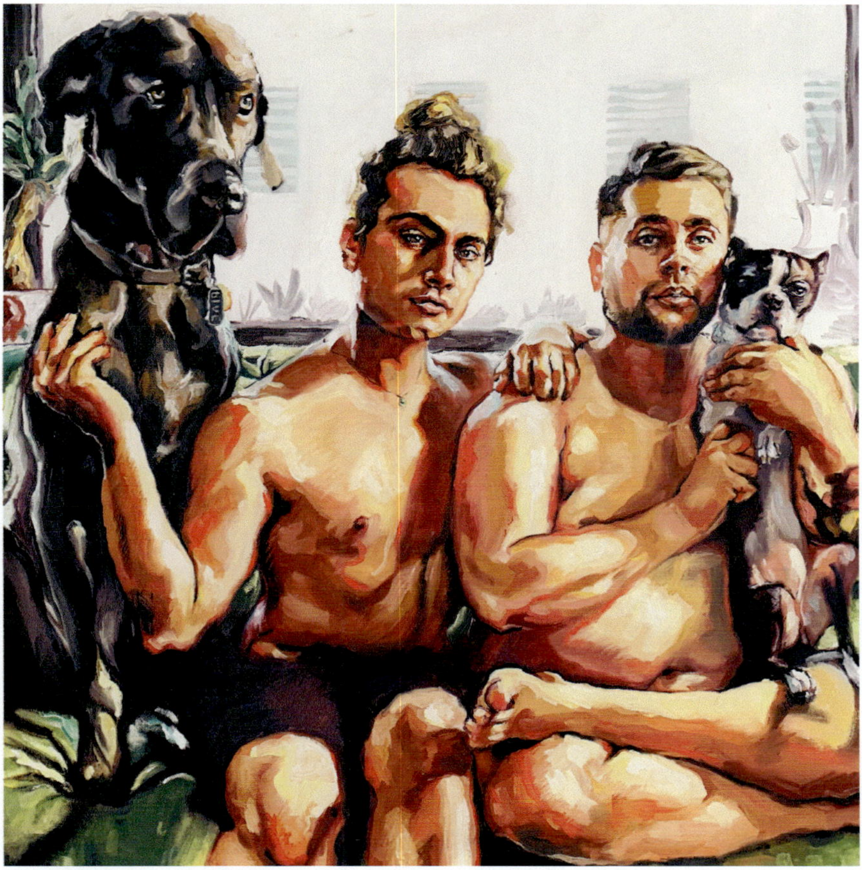

***Figure 7.1*** *"Queer Family Portrait," by Zachary D. Van Den Berg.*

*Note*: Oil on linen, 36 × 36 inches. This painting depicts the author's family seated on a chartreuse velour couch in front of a window, with gestural marks suggesting potted plants and a vase of flowers. From left to right: Blue, the Great Dane; the author; their partner, Rocco; and Stella, the Boston Terrier.

The culmination of this exploration was a solo exhibition at one of the galleries at the Center on Halsted, one of Chicago's largest LGBTQIA+ community centers, held just before commencing my master's coursework in art therapy and counseling. The exhibit featured eight queer family portraits of my friends and loved ones, each painted with love and care and later donated to the families. Almost all the families depicted attended the opening reception, proud to be part of the exhibit (Figure 7.2).

This exhibition represented not merely a personal milestone but also a dialogic space that bridged my own experiences with the broader,

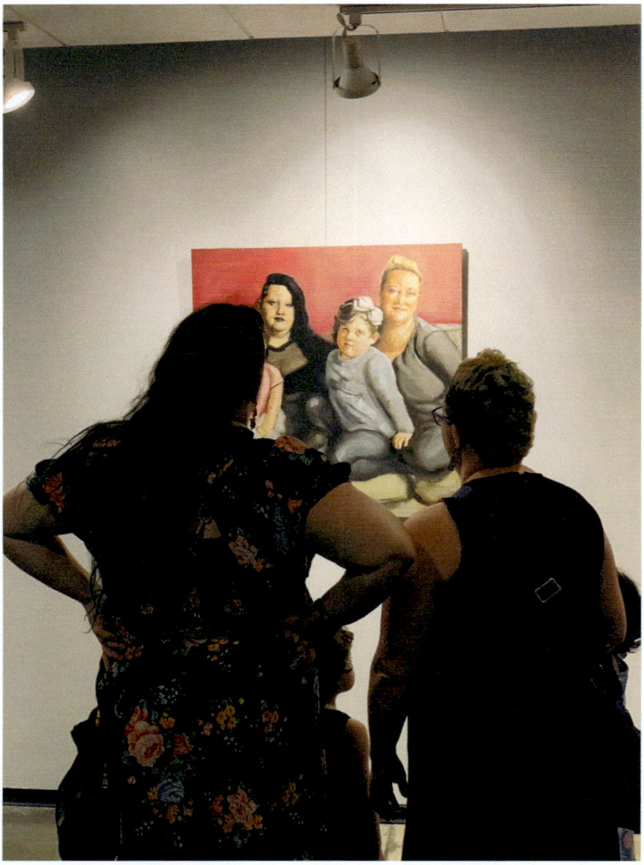

*Figure 7.2* *Opening Reception, "Queer Family Portraits," 2019.*

*Note*: Two parents viewing their portrait displayed at the Center on Halsted Gallery during the opening reception of the exhibit.

historical trajectories of LGBTQIA+ kinship-building networks. Through this sustained artistic inquiry, I was able to understand myself within a rich lineage of queer existence and resistance, embracing the abundant possibilities, care, and love that define our communities.

## EARLY EXPERIENCES IN ART THERAPY EDUCATION

When I began working on my master's degree, I was met with a dissonance between the anticipation of engaging deeply with art therapy—particularly its intersections with queer art activism and LGBTQIA+ community care practices—and the reality of the formal curriculum. Courses that professed to delve into the history and theory of art therapy in the United States notably omitted queer narratives, overlooked the politics of mental health, and failed to address the intricate intersections of identity and difference. This omission posited an unsettling implication: that professional proficiency and ethical practice necessitated the marginalization of nondominant perspectives, insinuating that the acknowledgment of such identities might detract from the quality of client care.

The lack of LGBTQIA+ representation within student-accessible spheres, in the university and profession more broadly, amplified a sense of alienation, confronting me with pervasive cis-heteronormativity and the consequent marginalization of queer experiences, which have been noted by others (Van Den Berg, 2024; Zappa, 2017). This conventional orientation within art therapy discourse left me longing for a lineage of queer art therapists who had successfully integrated their personal and professional identities—a lineage notably absent. My engagement with queer theory and the exploration of my own sexual and gender identities in the context of academic pursuits underscored the challenge of finding communal spaces within the art therapy domain that resonated with these reflections. Encounters with resistance, ranging from subtle hesitancy to explicit shaming for broaching queerness in theoretical, historical, and clinical discussions, highlighted the prevailing tensions among peers and professionals. Despite these challenges, my commitment to feeling my way to community remained undeterred.

Propelled by a deep-seated desire for belonging and resonance within a community of shared queer experience, I sought out online art therapy communities where I could engage in meaningful dialogues. This pursuit of digital camaraderie with LGBTQIA+-identified art therapists and allies yielded enriching conversations, providing insights, wisdom, and invaluable resources from a diverse array of scholars, practitioners, educators, and peers. These interactions, replete with recurring themes and profound insights, illuminated the transformative potential of incorporating queer perspectives into art therapy. They underscored the necessity for the discipline to adopt more inclusive and diverse curricular and professional practices.

## DEVELOPING "INVISIBLE HISTORIES: THE LIVES AND WORKS OF LGBTQIA+ ART THERAPISTS" VIDEO SERIES

In collaboration with the support of Judy Rubin, I began to actively amplify the narratives of LGBTQIA+ art therapists through the creation of the "Invisible Histories" video series (Van Den Berg, 2020b). This endeavor began with honing my video-editing skills, spurred by Judy's encouragement. I established an interview framework and drafted a preliminary consent form. The dissemination of the videos exceeded my initial expectations, as participants referred the project on and also underscored the project's community-building potential, especially pronounced during the peak of quarantine when digital platforms like Zoom became vital tools for connection.

I adopted a collaborative development process, working with interviewees on the editing and revisions and continually sought out interviewee feedback. This approach not only ensured authentic representation of participants' narratives but also emphasized the importance of meaningful relationships in the storytelling process. We prioritized accessibility and incorporated closed captions, which underscored the series' educational potential, facilitating its integration into diverse classroom settings.

My dissemination strategy targeted online forums dedicated to social justice and transformative action within creative arts therapies, leading to affirmative community feedback that validated the project's direction and impact (Van Den Berg, 2020a). With over 1,500 video streams and 8,600 video impressions globally, the series has made significant inroads in raising awareness and fostering inclusivity within the profession. However, the search for queer-specific forums within creative arts therapies highlighted the ongoing need for spaces that address the intersectionality of LGBTQIA+ art therapists, underscoring the series' role in bridging this gap.

## FORMING THE COALITION FOR QUEER CREATIVE ARTS THERAPIES

In response to the absence of dedicated spaces for queer representation within creative arts therapies, I founded the Coalition for Queer Creative Arts Therapies in 2020, initially named Queer Creative Arts Therapies. This initiative was sparked by a spontaneous decision to leverage social media as a platform for community building, starting with a Facebook page. Drawing upon the ethos of existing groups for inspiration, I delineated the Coalition's mission to focus on queer arts therapies organization, resource dissemination, and the cultivation of a supportive community. Inviting individuals from my existing network, I aimed to foster broader participation and engagement.

The group's rapid expansion, over the course of a year amassing over a thousand members, underscored the pressing need for such a space within the creative arts therapies community. This growth not only reflected the Coalition's potential to serve as a pivotal resource and community for queer therapists, educators, students, and practitioners but also highlighted the transformative power of collective efforts in extending support and visibility beyond the digital confines of a Facebook forum.

## THE EMERGENCE OF EXPRESSING PRIDE

I was a volunteer with Expressive Media, Inc. (EMI) and the Expressive Therapies Summit when I proposed a collaboration with the Summit founder Barry Cohen: organizing a dedicated virtual program within the Summit framework, coinciding with Pride month, to showcase LGBTQIA+ expressive arts methodologies. The vision was to document these sessions for inclusion in the EMI Film Library, thereby extending the reach and impact of queer-affirming principles across the arts therapy disciplines. Barry insightfully suggested the event's orchestration through our Facebook group, with co-sponsorship by the Summit and Arte Terapia en Espanol (an art therapy organization connecting practitioners across Latin America), thereby leveraging the Coalition's visibility and resources while marking its foray into professional development.

The all-day virtual program featured bilingual translation and brought together facilitators from around the world to explore diverse LGBTQIA+ topics in creative arts therapies, each rooted in regional expressions of queerness. The online platform allowed participants to join and leave at their convenience, with the assurance that all presentations were recorded and available for later streaming. Participants actively engaged through the chat feature, fostering a dynamic exchange of questions, interests, and appreciation. This interaction facilitated the sharing of resources, ideas, and valuable information, demonstrating a community dedicated to accessibility and professional growth. The event was a powerful testament to the collective care and commitment within the community.

Through the inaugural Expressing Pride program (C-QCAT, 2024a), I gained valuable insights into copywriting, outreach strategies, presenter requisites, event planning logistics, and the crafting of engaging promotional material. The event's positive reception reaffirmed my belief in its transformative potential as a platform for community engagement, knowledge dissemination, and appreciation of the significant contributions LGBTQIA+ art therapists make to our communities. Nearly 300 registered from across the globe, and we had 50–80 people in attendance throughout the virtual program. The attendee post-event survey feedback underscored a collective desire for more: more sessions, more speakers, more topics, and requests for the development of a future in-person iteration.

As Expressing Pride approached its second year (C-QCAT, 2024b), I drew on the invaluable lessons and mentorship from Barry, the Summit team, and EMI. I wanted to push my boundaries by taking on a more independent role in programming this iteration. While I was committed to ensuring that Expressing Pride would eventually have multiple leaders from our LGBTQIA+ communities in creative arts therapies, I found myself conflicted. Despite my aspiration, I was not yet ready to fully relinquish control. I struggled with embracing the vulnerability and courage needed for decentralized leadership and relying on others for a project so close to my heart.

## LEARNING FROM FAILURES

Despite the encouraging success marked by enthusiastic participation and positive feedback, a reflective examination reveals the inherent limitations and ethical concerns associated with a leadership model overly reliant on a single person. I offer this not only as an exercise in practicing humility in the face of failure but also as a critical self-reflexive exploration of how unexamined social privileges can subtly influence and potentially undermine the collective efforts essential for community-oriented endeavors.

The program's operational effectiveness, underscored by my sole leadership for content curation and event facilitation, inadvertently marginalized the inclusive and transformative potential of community-centered planning. This realization emerged from confronting the dual challenges of resource scarcity and my hesitance to lead and delegate effectively. This recognition was compounded by a fear of the vulnerability associated with asking and receiving help, and led to discord between my aspirations for Expressing Pride and its realized approach. This dissonance not only contributed to burnout and mental health challenges for me but also highlighted the necessity for a leadership model that emphasizes mutuality, radical care, and decentralization.

Attendee feedback illuminated the benefits of distributed responsibilities and the potential for collaborative efforts to alleviate workload pressures. Such insights signal the critical need for a paradigm shift toward a more sustainable and inclusive approach to the project, one that resonates with the ethos of grassroots queer activism and coalition-building. The recalibration of my leadership within Expressing Pride and subsequent initiatives reflects my growing awareness of the value of vulnerability, humility, and the reciprocal exchange of support within the community. By advocating for broader community support and decentralized leadership, this approach aims not only to mitigate burnout but also to ensure the continuity and vitality of community-centric programs, embodying the collective action necessary for humble community endeavors.

## ADAPTATIONS FROM THESE LESSONS

As Expressing Pride progressed into its third year, in 2023, the program underwent a significant transformation, embodying the invaluable insights gleaned from its formative phases. This evolution was marked by a deliberate shift toward a model of communal collaboration and collective wisdom, underscoring the power of community engagement in driving the program's mission. The catalyst for this strategic pivot was an outreach initiative for volunteers, executed through the Coalition's social media platforms, which garnered an immediate and enthusiastic response from the community. The inaugural volunteer meeting served as a critical juncture of connection, understanding, and collective envisioning, where participants shared personal stories, deliberated on the symposium's future direction, and identified individual contributions toward its growth.

This gathering signaled a pivotal shift toward harnessing our community's collective intelligence, culminating in a consensus on the adoption of promising new organizational structures, equitable workload distribution, decentralized decision-making, and clear role delineations. The formation of committees—programming, outreach, marketing, and logistics/IT—epitomized our commitment to a collaborative operational workflow, fostering a sense of interconnectivity and mutual support essential for the program's logistical and creative undertakings.

In anticipation of the first meeting with volunteers, I meticulously reviewed all the documentation from the program's inception to its most recent iteration to ensure everyone would have all the information available up to that point. This endeavor was instrumental in consolidating and organizing administrative content in alignment with our collaborative planning ethos. This meticulous preparation ensured that every volunteer received a comprehensive understanding of the program's historical context and operational framework, thus fostering an environment characterized by transparency and inclusivity from the onset.

The collective stewardship of Expressing Pride 2023 underscored the community's capacity for grace, discernment, and adaptability, vital to solidifying the program's annual presence within the Coalition and the wider community (C-QCAT, 2024c). This concerted effort was not only aimed at preserving the symposium's foundational objectives but also at enhancing its commitment to fostering critical knowledge and support for queer-affirming practices across the creative arts therapies.

## OUTCOMES FROM THE ADAPTATIONS

Expressing Pride 2023 serves as a reminder of the power of collective effort and the significant impact of community-driven initiatives, marking a transition from an individual endeavor to a shared journey of profession-building, place-making, and sustainability. The resoundingly positive feedback from attendees marked the event a success, and an "inclusive," "hopeful," and "transformative space" for learning. Such generous survey responses reflect the deep appreciation for the team's dedication to creating an accessible and niche educational experience for both professionals and students.

In anticipation of the growing needs of our community and with the goal of expanding the reach of Expressing Pride, we developed a website to serve as a repository for recorded presentations. This digital archive is composed of dozens of sessions that encompass the breadth of creative arts therapies from a queer-affirming perspective; it has become an invaluable resource for practitioners, educators, and students, facilitating ongoing learning and collaboration. This initiative underscores the symposium's dedication to promoting practices that are both affirming and generative, which has not gone unnoticed by other organizations.

As we navigated the transition toward formal incorporation as a nonprofit, our initiative encountered significant financial challenges. Despite the absence of a monetary reserve for the funding of the website or the development of additional resources, the team's creative ingenuity shone through. By using free online tools and strategically leveraging platforms such as Google Sites and YouTube, we devised a solution that not only protected our content but also ensured its accessibility to those committed to our mission. This strategy highlights our dedication to maximizing the availability of resources while we explore opportunities for financial growth and the enhancement of our services.

## RECENT DEVELOPMENTS

The generosity of the European Federation of Art Therapy (EFAT) in sharing relevant LGBTQIA+ recorded content with the Coalition for free is a meaningful development in our mission to foster an inclusive and supportive professional environment (C-QCAT, 2024d). This collaboration not only enriches our repository of resources but also underscores our collective aspiration to establish the Coalition as a reliable, respected, and recognized repository for LGBTQIA+ continuing education and professional development within the creative arts therapies. The EFAT's contribution exemplifies the transformative power of interorganizational partnerships in expanding access to critical educational materials, thereby supporting the ongoing growth and empowerment of practitioners committed to queer-affirming practices.

In addition, efforts are underway to navigate the procedural landscape required to attain accreditation as a continuing education provider for the National Board for Certified Counselors. This endeavor, aimed at offering complimentary and flexible pay-as-you-can continuing education (CE) credits, signifies our dedication to the ongoing professional development of those engaging with our resources. The forthcoming year marks a milestone with the offering of CE-eligible presentations at no cost, thanks to the support and co-sponsorship of Creative Wellbeing Workshops, LLC. This partnership, involving the generosity of Gioia Chilton and Rebecca Wilkinson, exemplifies the profound impact of resource sharing, active allyship, and community care in realizing our collective aspirations for professional inclusivity.

Taken together, it is our shared vision that these collaborations will continue and lead to more partnerships with other organizations in the future. Such noncompetitive and mutually beneficial relationships ensure that everyone's needs are equitably met with care. By actively seeking and humbly fostering such interorganizational collaborations, we aim to enhance the accessibility and diversity of educational content available to creative arts therapists worldwide. This strategic approach not only strengthens the professional capacities of individual practitioners but also contributes to the broader effort to create a more inclusive, affirming, and supportive environment for LGBTQIA+ clients and communities within the realm of creative arts therapies.

Lastly, with the official recognition of the Coalition as a nonprofit organization in the state of Texas and national tax-exempt status as a 501(c)(3) entity, we are laying the groundwork for financial sustainability and broader fundraising capabilities. Importantly, this transition ushers in a decentralized governance model, characterized by a board of directors actively engaged in shared responsibilities and decision-making. This structural shift reinforces our commitment to transparency, collaborative leadership, and the core values of community-driven initiatives and equity, paving the way for a future where Expressing Pride continues to flourish.

## CLOSING REFLECTIONS

The journey undertaken by the Coalition and Expressing Pride represents a profound exploration into the realms of vulnerability, humility, and the transformative power of community support. These reflections serve to underscore the essential roles of inclusivity and communal connectedness as beacons that have guided my path, illuminating uncharted territories in both my personal and professional landscapes. The enthusiastic reception of and support for these initiatives indicate a widespread and collective yearning within the LGBTQIA+ community and its allies for spaces that affirm and celebrate queer identities within the creative arts therapies field.

This shared aspiration for recognition and authentic communal connection reflects the broader narrative of LGBTQIA+ experiences, characterized by sexual and gender marginalization and enriched by a profound sense of interconnectedness and kinship. Contrary to initial apprehensions, this nexus of mutual experiences has not posed a professional barrier but has acted as a bridge, fostering enhanced ethical introspection, self-awareness, and transformative practice. The inherent solidarity and kinship within our community offers a unique lens for deeper understanding and empathy, challenging and enriching professional ethics rather than complicating them.

As articulated in this reflection, queer kinship transcends mere relational ties, embodying a profound ethic of care that defines how LGBTQIA+ and allied creative arts therapists relate to ourselves, each other, our clients, and the creative process. This ethos nurtures mutual flourishing across various communities, inviting us to tap into a wellspring of transgenerational wisdom, resilience, and strength. Engaging with this interconnectedness situates us within the vibrant cultural tapestry of queerness, not simply as a reconnection with history but as active participants in shaping a present that lays the groundwork for future generations. This engagement fosters a landscape ripe for justice and potentiality, making the creation of more queer worlds not just a possibility but a reality.

Through these collective endeavors, we affirm the power of community-driven initiatives to transform and enrich the field of creative arts therapies, championing queer-affirming practices, and the creation of inclusive spaces that honor the diversity and richness of queer identities and experiences.

## ACKNOWLEDGMENTS

I would like to share my deepest gratitude to every volunteer who has and continues to support the Coalition and its annual offering, Expressing Pride. I would like to thank my fellow Board of Directors of C-QCAT: Sara Blevins-Ranes, Sharon Arbtin, Nicolas Denson, and Rachel Van Den Berg.

## REFERENCES

Anderson, M. (2020). Queer ethos in art therapy. In L. Leone (Ed.), *Craft in art therapy: Diverse approaches to the transformative power of craft materials and methods* (pp. 218–236). Routledge.

*Coalition for Queer Creative Arts Therapies—2021.* (2024a). Expressing Pride 2021. Retrieved from www.coalitionforqueercats.org/expressing-pride/2021

*Coalition for Queer Creative Arts Therapies—2022.* (2024b). Expressing Pride 2022. Retrieved from www.coalitionforqueercats.org/expressing-pride/2022

*Coalition for Queer Creative Arts Therapies—2023.* (2024c). Expressing Pride 2023. Retrieved from www.coalitionforqueercats.org/expressing-pride/2023

*Coalition for Queer Creative Arts Therapies—2024.* (2024d). Single Sessions. Retrieved from www.coalitionforqueercats.org/expressing-pride/single-sessions

DeLucia, J., Mikel, E., Lombardi, R., Nolan, E., Dejkameh, M., & Davis, C. (2020). *The act of creation: Art therapist as entrepreneur* [Panel presentation]. American Therapy Association 51st Annual Conference.

DeLucia, J., Royster, R., Lounsbury, L., Andrus, M., & Stallings, J. (2021). *Creative change agent: Therapist as entrepreneur* [Panel presentation]. American Therapy Association 51st Annual Conference.

Hetherington, R. (2020). Invisible complicity in LGBTQI art therapy: A series of case studies in response to Hadley's call for the need for vigilance. *The Arts in Psychotherapy, 70*(2), 101667–101669. https://doi.org/10.1016/j.aip.2020.101667

Newey, L. R. (2017). "Changing the system": Compensatory versus transformative social entrepreneurship. *Journal of Social Entrepreneurship, 9*(1), 1–18. https://doi.org/10.1080/19420676.2017.1408671

Talwar, S. (2015). Creating alternative public spaces: Community-based art practice, critical consciousness and social justice. In D. Gussak & M. Rosal (Eds.), *The Wiley-Blackwell handbook of art therapy* (pp. 840–847). Wiley Blackwell.

Van Den Berg, Z. D. (2020a, November 16). *Illuminating "invisible histories" of LGBTQ+ art therapists.* Adler University Stories. Retrieved from www.adler.edu/2020/11/16/illuminating-invisible-histories-of-lgbtq-art-therapists/

Van Den Berg, Z. D. (2020b). *Invisible histories: The lives and works of LGBTQ+ art therapists* [Video Series]. Retrieved from https://vimeo.com/showcase/7642762

Van Den Berg, Z. D. (2023). Proposing an ar(t)chive of queer forms with sexual, gender, and relationship diverse clients. *Art Therapy: Journal of the American Art Therapy Association, 41*(1), 44–50. https://doi.org/10.1080/07421656.2023.2240677

Van Den Berg, Z. D. (2024). Opinion piece: Addressing traumatic experiences of cis-heterosexism with LGBTQIA+ clients in art therapy. *International Journal of Art Therapy, 29*(1), 1–10. https://doi.org/10.1080/17454832.2023.2261542

Van Den Berg, Z. D., & Anderson, M. (2023). Queer worldmaking in sex-positive art therapy: Radical strategies for individual healing and social transformation. *Art Therapy: Journal of the American Art Therapy Association, 40*(4), 188–196. https://doi.org/10.1080/07421656.2023.2193660

Zappa, A. (2017). Beyond erasure: The ethics of art therapy research with trans and gender-independent people. *Art Therapy, 34*(3), 129–134. https://doi.org/10.1080/07421656.2017.1343074

*Chapter* **8**

# Social Entrepreneurship in Licensure and Educational Advocacy

*Jessica Woolhiser Stallings, Jenelle Miller, Yasmin Henderson, and Jennifer Jividen Jackson*

Nebraska has few art therapists and no graduate training programs in art therapy. However, on January 1, 2025, Nebraska became the first central U.S. state with an art therapy–specific license. Until then, art therapists who sought licensing were sometimes considered as members of a counseling field. However, there was no guarantee that art therapists would be approved for a counseling license, and they often had to complete educational requirements in addition to their art therapy master's degree to qualify. This lack of state-level regulation left Nebraskans vulnerable to harm from unqualified providers. The Nebraska Art Therapy Licensure Coalition (NATLC) was formed to address these issues and consists of our chapter authors. This chapter discusses the formation of the NATLC and its advocacy and work toward licensure regulation in the state of Nebraska and provides practical tips based on NATLC's experience.

## IDENTIFYING OPPORTUNITY

In 2016, Jenelle Miller, a founding member of the NATLC, went to the American Art Therapy Association (AATA) annual conference and spoke with the association about how to establish a graduate-level training program in art therapy in Nebraska. This inquiry emerged as a result of a barrier Jenelle and others in the state identified. Although Jenelle received her undergraduate pre-art therapy degree and master's degree in social work in Nebraska, specific graduate-level training in art therapy was unavailable in the state. Since such education is a requirement for becoming a registered and board-certified art therapist, art therapists could not practice within the state unless they received their education elsewhere. Trained art therapists

DOI: 10.4324/9781032615776-9

often did not return to practice in the state, resulting in a lack of art therapy services available to Nebraskans. AATA's executive director suggested that developing licensure in the state was the first step, and then graduate programs could be established to keep local art therapy students in Nebraska.

Art therapy has long fought for recognition as a field equivalent to social work and counseling. Recognition of art therapy as a distinct mental health profession is complicated as many art therapists across the country receive licensure under allied professions. Nebraska has traditionally regarded art therapy as part of the counseling field, with licensure only attainable through mental health counseling standards. As discussed, this structure excludes some trained in art therapy from licensing, as not all art therapy education aligns with counseling's educational standards. This also leads to challenges in educating others about the similarities and differences between art therapy and other mental health fields, as the licensure structure itself implied that art therapy was not an independent field with educational standards and practice theories of its own.

Most importantly, licensure or certification is important to provide enforceable standards of practice to protect citizens. Lacking this, anyone can state that they are providing art therapy services regardless of their training. If the state recognizes art therapist as a professional title using a regulated license or certification, it reduces the potential for harm and increases the availability of services.

Jenelle's initial inquiry in 2016 led to the formation of the Nebraska Art Therapy Licensure Coalition (NATLC) and the pursuit of an art therapy–specific credential in Nebraska. Pursuing art therapy–specific credentialing would result in legally defining the similarities and differences between art therapy and counseling. This came with an inherent risk of art therapy being dropped entirely from licensure eligibility if the bill was not successful. Despite this risk, NATLC decided to go forward as we felt the benefits outweighed the risks.

The following sections provide an overview of our experience and practical tips for legislative advocacy. Although each state has its own process, the necessary content areas, supporting information, social capital, and social entrepreneurial skills to promote success are the same.

## ACHIEVING LICENSURE IN NEBRASKA

### Social Capital, Entrepreneurship, and Extrapreneurship

Social capital refers to the building and use of relationships for networking, leading to personal, professional, and community gains (Putnam, 1994).

It is an essential ingredient in social entrepreneurship and extrapreneurship. Social entrepreneurs facilitate system change by creating ventures that benefit society (Alvord et al., 2004). Social extrapreneurs work across organizations to facilitate change, often in structures where they are not formal members or employees (van Rooijen, 2017). Social capital provides the foundational relationships for these endeavors.

Jenelle exercised social entrepreneurship in initiating the art therapy licensure bill. After discussing the lack of graduate education and licensure in art therapy in Nebraska with the AATA's executive director, she reached out to "Nebraskans For the Arts" (NFTA), a nonprofit arts advocacy agency. NFTA is an organization affiliated with Americans for the Arts that promotes arts-based agendas in the Nebraska political sector. Jenelle participated in a three-month volunteer internship with NFTA, learning how to establish a bill for art therapy licensure in Nebraska.

Simultaneously, Jessica was working on a doctoral degree in art therapy and investigating the potential for creating a graduate-level art therapy degree in Nebraska. Jessica connected with Jenelle through Jennifer Jividen Jackson, an art therapist and executive director of Heartland Counseling Services in South Sioux City Nebraska, and became a signatory on the NATLC request for a sunrise review to initiate a licensure bill.

Yasmin Henderson was brought into the NATLC by Jessica. Yasmin's expertise in professional networking and private practice proved essential to our efforts. Each of us used social capital in our professional relationships to advocate for our licensure proposal, gain the support of key partners, and employed extrapreneurship to bring together the resources of organizations that supported our initiative.

Extrapreneurship played a vital role in our success as a small group of art therapists advocating for state-wide legislation changes. Partnering with NFTA was essential in sustaining the movement for art therapist certification and licensure in Nebraska. In 2018, Doug Zbylut, the NFTA executive director, believed in the bill and helped the coalition begin the steps to advocate for legislative change. Our first NATLC meeting was held at the NFTA offices on July 26, 2018, with Doug, Jenelle, Jennifer, and Nebraska art therapist Pamela Muggenberg and art therapy students Lindsey Hylen and Hannah Rose [Walsh]. Doug approached Senator Sara Howard to sponsor the bill, and she agreed. After her term ended, our team needed to find a new sponsor for the bill. Jennifer Jividen Jackson approached her senator, Republican Joni Albrecht, who agreed to sponsor the bill and continues to work with NATLC.

After Doug Zbylut's retirement in 2020, we worked with the interim Executive Director Skyler Dykes, followed by Executive Director Petra

Wahlqvist (2021–2023). In 2023, Dr. Lance Nielsen assumed the executive director role and assisted the NATLC in the final push for passage of the bill. Without NFTA, we would not have been able to get the bill passed. NFTA has provided advocacy and lobbying at no cost, which was essential in advancing this legislation.

In addition to NFTA, developing community with allied professionals was essential. As extrapreneurs we continued to reach out to other organizations and professionals to establish connections and access to resources that would further our efforts. For instance, Dr. Susan Reay, a social work professor, initially became acquainted with the NATLC as a member of the mental health licensing board for Nebraska. The Mental Health Board, as led by Dr. Reay, articulated that they did not support the bill as they believed art therapy was not an independent field with independent theories, making art therapy a technique or modality rather than a profession, leading to a delay in its passage. Following this, Dr. Reay invited Yasmin to guest speak at the University of Nebraska Omaha at their Entrepreneurship Day and they began to build a relationship that supported professional understanding, mutual curiosity, and respect. After this, Dr. Reay became a supporter of the bill. The Mental Health Board also dropped their objections.

## Nebraska's Legislative Process

Nebraska has a long history of legislative uniqueness, perhaps best known for the splitting of its electoral college votes in presidential elections. This uniqueness also includes the structure of our legislature and the processes for certifying and licensing mental health professionals. Nebraska's unique governing structure and licensure process provide important context for understanding NATLC, our work, and the necessity of social entrepreneurship and creative advocacy. The state legislature is the only single-house legislature in the United States, referred to as the Unicameral. This consists of a Senate chamber. The people of Nebraska are often referred to as the "second house" and citizen committees and public votes have a large role in state government.

### *Nebraska Sunrise Review*

In the case of mental health and other health-related licensure issues, the second house is represented by a Sunrise Review process where a citizen committee reviews an extensive proposal and holds public hearings to determine the necessity and viability of licensure requests. This is initiated after a bill draft is submitted by the bill's sponsor, a member of the Senate who has agreed to and/or initiated the bill. In this review, four criteria are to be met to justify furthering the process. These include:

> *Criterion 1*: Unregulated practice can clearly harm or endanger the health, safety, or welfare of the public.
>
> *Criterion 2*: Regulation of the profession does not impose significant new economic hardship on the public, significantly diminish the supply of qualified practitioners, or otherwise create barriers to service that are not consistent with the public welfare and interest.
>
> *Criterion 3*: The public needs assurance from the state of initial and continuing professional ability.
>
> *Criterion 4*: The public cannot be protected by a more effective alternative. (Nebraska Department of Health and Human Services, 2021)

To meet these four criteria, the NATLC provided detailed responses to 29 questions about the applicant group (NATLC) and the proposal for state regulation of art therapy by creating a path toward discipline-specific licensure through the state's licensure and credentialing structure. These questions addressed areas such as identifying stakeholders inside and outside the profession, agencies, and other settings where the profession may work, credentialing already in place, other ways the profession may be regulated and whether they are sufficient, risk of harm due to lack of licensure, economic burden or benefit, and included letters of support from stakeholders and places of employment. Our proposal submitted for review was 187 pages (Nebraska Art Therapy Licensure Coalition, 2019).

In general practice, after the Sunrise Review Committee reviews and approves the proposal, it moves on to the Nebraska Department of Health and Human Services (DHHS) for approval. If DHHS approves the proposal, a bill then proceeds to the legislature's Health and Human Services Committee. At this stage, it receives another public hearing, and the committee decides if it will come to a floor vote. In our case, the NATLC's bill passed at the committee level three times and two of these times failed to go to a floor vote. The first time the bill failed to reach a floor vote was due to premature closure of the session due to COVID-19 pandemic restrictions. The second time it failed due to opposition from the state mental health board. Our third and successful attempt to move the bill through to a vote was in the 2023–2024 legislative session and is detailed near the end of this chapter.

*Mental Health Licensing Structure*

Nebraska has an unusual mental health licensing structure, where most mental health professions are eligible for licensure as a Licensed Mental Health Practitioner (LMHP) or Licensed Independent Mental Health Practitioner (LIMHP) rather than obtaining a discipline-specific license. In addition to licensure, professionals certify in their individual discipline at the state level. For example, the statute allows for an LMHP or an LIMHP who certifies in marriage and family therapy to be called a Licensed Marriage and Family Therapist (see Figure 8.1), thus indirectly providing discipline-specific licensure (State of Nebraska, 2022).

The NATLC initially proposed a full art therapy licensure bill, but the Sunrise Review Committee process determined that we should instead ask for the existing Mental Health Practice Act statute to be opened and for art therapy certification language to be added. Our bill was initially introduced in 2019 and then sent to the Sunrise Review Committee, after approval at that level and from the Nebraska DHHS, the revised bill was introduced again in 2021. In the 2021–2022 legislative session, we met opposition from the mental health licensing board arguing that art therapy was not an independent profession but rather a technique used by the other mental health disciplines. In the 2023–2024 session, there were no objections from the licensure board. NFTA was instrumental in compiling

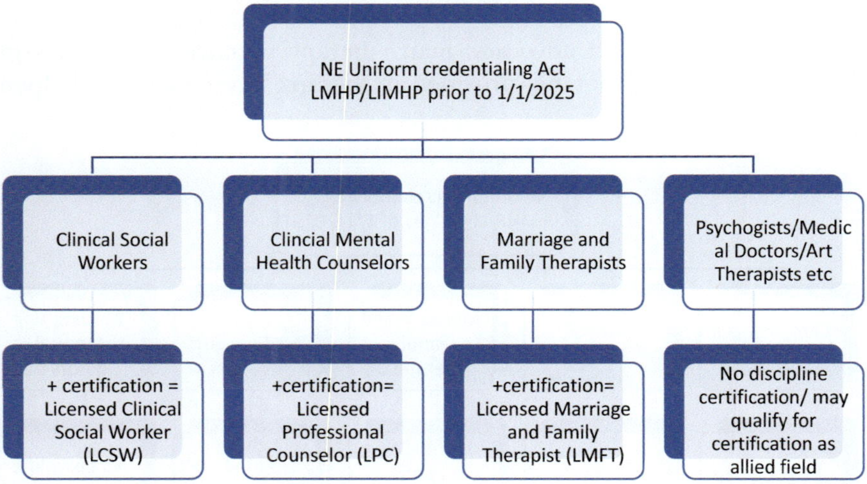


***Figure 8.1*** *Nebraska Uniform Credentialing Act Prior to Passage of Licensure Bill 605*

the Sunrise Review Report and providing feedback on the initial bill drafts and subsequent edits. They also assisted with lobbying and testified before committees alongside Nebraska art therapists.

## PASSAGE OF THE BILL

The Legislative Bill 605 (hereinafter "LB 605") passed out of committee in February 2023, after Jessica Woolhiser Stallings (on behalf of Heartland Family Service), Petra Wahlquist, and Senator Albrecht testified before the Health and Human Services Committee of the Unicameral. LB 605 came up for a vote in the second half of the legislative session in February 2024, when it passed the first and second of three floor votes moving it through the unicameral process. At this time, LB 605 gained a second sponsor, Democratic Senator George Dungan III. In March 2024, Nebraska LB 605, which revises the Nebraska Uniform Credentialing Act, was passed unanimously by the Nebraska Unicameral. The bill was subsequently signed by Governor Jim Pillen (Nebraska Legislature, n.d.; Nebraska Legislature, 2024).

The provisions of the bill providing art therapy credentialing and licensure became effective January 1, 2025 (see Figure 8.2), making Nebraska the thirteenth state/territory with an art therapy–specific license in the United States. As of writing this in August 2024, Nebraska is the only state in the Great Plains region with art therapy licensure (American Art Therapy Association, n.d.).

### Protection of the Public Through Licensure

Prior to licensure and advocacy, many therapy practices and artists in Nebraska advertised that they provided art therapy. These examples helped

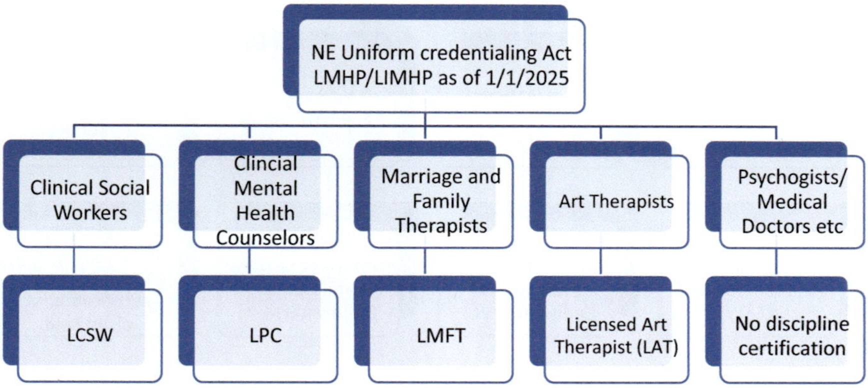


***Figure 8.2*** *Nebraska Uniform Credentialing Act After the Passage of Licensure Bill 605*

to provide justification for specific licensure. Without licensure, art therapy was entirely unregulated by the state, increasing the risk of harm for clients. Harm to the public was the most salient element of the four criteria mentioned previously in justifying the initiation of a new license in the state of Nebraska. Three of the four criteria mentioned the need to protect the public or to assure quality of services to the public. Although the four members of NATLC were dually qualified art therapists by having professional training in art therapy and meeting the qualifications for counseling licensure, many people who state they provide art therapy in the state of Nebraska do not have art therapy–specific training. Continuing to operate without art therapy–specific licensure jeopardized the sustainability of the practice within the state due to inconsistency in the care provided. This left the public vulnerable to receiving services from someone with no mental health training or working with a mental health professional without knowledge of the specific harms that can be caused when using art materials without knowledge of their possible psychological impacts.

This was perhaps best described by the director of Nebraska DHHS in his letter to the Unicameral, given as follows:

> Under the current practice situation of art therapy in Nebraska anyone may set up a practice as an art therapist and begin providing services to the public without having to satisfy any educational or training requirements to provide this kind of therapy. The applicants have documented that harm not only can occur as a result of this unregulated practice situation but that it actually has occurred as a result of this situation.
>
> The applicants' proposal would address this situation by requiring that those who seek to provide art therapy services satisfy all current Nebraska requirements for licensure as an LMHP before being allowed to provide this therapy. Additionally, no practitioner would be allowed to use the protected title of "Art Therapist" without satisfying both the LMHP requirement and satisfying additional requirements associated with becoming certified as an Art Therapist. However, a practitioner would not have to qualify to use the protected title in order to provide the services. LMHP status alone would allow a provider to provide art therapy services.
>
> (Anthone, 2020, p. 2)

A compromise was necessary in the passage of the bill. In an ideal world, we would have liked to restrict use of the term "art therapy" to those with specific training in art therapy. However, this was not acceptable to allied mental health fields. As a result, our bill was revised to state that in order to provide art therapy one must, at minimum, have training in a mental health field, and in order to call oneself and art therapist one must have specific art therapy training.

## PRACTICAL TIPS FROM OUR EFFORTS

### Leveraging Social Capital

Each member of NATLC has their own connections and social capital that have contributed to the sustainability and success of the NATLC's advocacy efforts. All four of us have worked to increase the accessibility of art therapy in the communities we serve while working toward licensing. This work was essential because demonstrating the viability of art therapy services, even without a specific license, provided support for its licensure and demonstrated a need for state regulation.

Yasmin built a thriving private practice, demonstrating the demand for art therapy services. Jessica and Jenelle developed art therapy programs at existing local agencies, reaching underserved populations and integrating art therapy into community mental health initiatives. Jennifer, as the executive director of a mental health agency prioritized hiring art therapists, increasing employment opportunities, and demonstrating the value of art therapy within established mental health programs.

The social capital we gained from the development of these programs has been crucial to our social entrepreneurship in achieving licensure. For example, our network of professional relationships helped us to effectively advocate with policymakers and gather community support. In addition, building these programs helped to highlight the necessity of establishing a license by illustrating high demand for art therapy services and the positive outcomes they produce.

### Teamwork

Teamwork is crucial when promoting grassroots causes, such as promoting art therapy's benefits on behalf of citizens who live in Nebraska. Teamwork provided the following benefits that were critical for us to build momentum in our effort to advocate for licensure in Nebraska and will assist you in yours:

*Strength in numbers:* Working together as a team made our efforts more powerful. When joining forces, we accomplished more than if we were working alone.

*Diverse skills and perspectives:* Everyone brought something valuable to the table. We all have different skills, experiences, and perspectives on art therapy, as well as differing experiences with licensure efforts in other states. This diversity allowed for a well-rounded approach to problem-solving and planning, ensuring that multiple aspects of our efforts were considered.

*Sharing the workload:* Changing legislation and passing new laws require a lot of work, from organizing meetings to spreading awareness. Tasks, trips, and testifying were divided among team members, making the workload more manageable for everyone. This helped prevent burnout and kept the momentum going for nearly seven years.

*Local knowledge:* In a rural state like Nebraska, local knowledge is invaluable—it is always who you know. This was particularly helpful when we had to find a senator to sponsor our bill. Building on established relationships has been helpful. Team members from different communities in Nebraska provided insights into the specific needs, challenges, and opportunities inherent to each area. This ensured that our efforts were tailored to the realities of the community.

*Amplifying voices:* The more people involved, the louder the message. Having team members from across the state allowed us to amplify our voice and reach a broader audience. This is especially important when trying to raise awareness or advocate for a cause in a rural setting where communication channels may be limited.

We thrived with teamwork and support of each other knowing our limits both personally and professionally. We encouraged each other to keep personal and professional balance to manage sustainability. This led to each of us stepping back when needed over the course of our efforts. We took turns leading the effort to make our coalition more resilient and successful. This engagement also assisted in sustaining our efforts, as we were all prepared to back each other up or take over at a moment's notice.

## Networking and Finding Allies

We networked by introducing ourselves to people in leadership positions. Each of us tends toward introversion, and we are all observers by nature. Our tendency toward introversion assisted in our efforts by allowing us to stand back and observe the needs of our key partners, interested parties, and ourselves in order to best structure our efforts to provide maximum benefit for all. We also had to break out of our natural tendency to watch and wait, and instead engage actively. Although this was more challenging for all of us, our dedication to our efforts and passion for our field and its accessibility to clients gave us the motivation to work through challenges. Our ability to rely on each other gave us strength in numbers which also helped sustain our efforts in networking. We recommend following a similar structure in your efforts.

Through our observations, research, and networking we found our best allies were those already focused on arts advocacy. Without the free advocacy work of NFTA and access to their resources, our small group would not have been able to sustain our efforts.

In addition, through the guidance of AATA and NFTA, we sought legislative sponsors who were already advocates for mental health and/or populations of people with which we often work. Our primary sponsor Senator Albrecht has a history of advocacy for mental health services. Knowing your legislators' priorities will help you identify who is most likely to work with you on licensure.

### Ask for More

A potentially counterintuitive piece of advice is to ask for more than you want or need. We started with a request for an art therapy license independent of the other professions. We then moved to requesting inclusion under the existing Uniform Credentialing Act. Finally, we accepted that to get licensure and title protection, we could not restrict use of the term art therapy. The existence of a protected title of Licensed Art Therapist makes clear who has specific training to provide art therapy.

### Identifying Essential Information

Although not all states have a Sunrise Review Process, the material required provides a guide to relevant information that legislators and other stakeholders will be seeking (see Nebraska Art Therapy Licensure Coalition, 2019, for example). Based on the requirements we recommend compiling a comprehensive list of art therapists in the state. This can be difficult to achieve as not all art therapists are formally credentialed. Resources that are helpful include the Art Therapy Credentials Board *find an art therapist* feature, sites such as Psychology Today where mental health professionals share profiles to obtain clients and contacting graduate programs who may be willing to contact graduates on your behalf about their inclusion in your list.

In addition to this list, compiling a list of the agencies that employ art therapists and other mental health professionals assists in identifying where the public may encounter these services. This list serves multiple purposes. It provides you a list of places to contact to seek letters of support, indicates where harm might occur if someone is practicing without proper training, and gives information on where art therapists may be employed in the future.

Engaging in meetings with your state's mental health board is also essential for answering questions about the advocacy effort and art therapy. The meetings are also a place where you will likely meet both opponents and supporters, allowing you to provide feedback to assist in your process.

Finally, and most importantly, you need to make a case that the public is at risk without licensure. If your state is like Nebraska, legislators are often reticent to impose more regulations and may even be anti-regulation. Therefore, you need to make a clear case that harm can occur from provision of services without enforceable regulations like those provided by licensure. If you have specific cases of harm you are familiar with from your state, those are the best to share; however, if you do not have examples from your region, contact other states and art therapy organizations like the American Art Therapy Association to obtain examples. We did not have specific harm cases in Nebraska; however, those provided by AATA from other states were sufficient to make our case. Although we may want licensure to increase job opportunities and job stability, the reason licensure exists is to protect the public.

## SUMMARY AND CONCLUSIONS

Over the course of 8 years, the key skills involved in social entrepreneurship were essential for all NATLC members. Forging relationships with various key partners and interested parties—including arts and mental health organizations, politicians, and other mental health and medical professionals—was crucial to the success of NATLC's bid for state licensure regulation. The NATLC provided countless hours of education to these various groups on the nuances of art therapy, the harm that could be caused due to lack of regulation, and the benefits of addressing provider shortages to meet the increasing demand for mental health services by expanding those qualified for mental health licensure in the state.

Art therapy licensure is a priority in many states. Our licensure bill was brought to passage through years of advocacy and relationship-building. Throughout, NFTA provided steadfast support, partnership, and assistance in developing and passing the legislation. Relationships with the state mental health board were adversarial in the beginning, but over time became cordial, and even in some cases turned into professional partnerships. The licensure bill gained supporters over the years, including universities, mental health agencies, individual providers, citizens of Nebraska, and Nebraska politicians. Bipartisan support was crucial in getting the bill passed.

Jenelle, Jennifer, Jessica, and Yasmin have all taken different paths in their art therapy careers but their combined experience and efforts along with a strong partnership with legislators, professionals, agencies, and NFTA supported the advancement of art therapy credentialing in our rural, low-population state. These efforts ensure protection of the public and sustainability of the profession in Nebraska.

We are now presented with two problems to address in Nebraska. Mental health therapies are generally paid for by third-party payers, most often insurance companies, but licensure does not ensure that services will be covered by these payers. Therefore, our next step in NATLC with NFTA is to lobby insurance panels to obtain reimbursement for the regulated practice of art therapy in Nebraska in order to make art therapists' services accessible to as many Nebraskans as possible. Ultimately, this also helps to address the originally identified problem of having graduate education availability within Nebraska, as it increases employment opportunities for art therapists, therefore making the profession a more viable option for those seeking to practice in a mental health field. We will continue working on these areas after a much-deserved self-care break.

## REFERENCES

Alvord, S. H., Brown, L. D., & Letts, C. W. (2004). Social entrepreneurship and societal transformation: An exploratory study. *Journal of Applied Behavioural Science, 40*, 260–282. https://doi.org/10.1177/0021886304266847

American Art Therapy Association. (n.d.). *State advocacy*. Retrieved from https://arttherapy.org/state-advocacy/

Anthone, G. J. (2020, May 6). *The director's report on the proposal to create a certification under LMHP for art therapists*. Department of Health and Human Services of Nebraska. Retrieved from https://dhhs.ne.gov/licensure/Credentialing%20Review%20Docs/CRArtTherDirReport.pdf

Nebraska Art Therapy Licensure Coalition. (2019). *Request for the credentialing review of art therapy*. Department of Health and Human Services of Nebraska. Retrieved from https://dhhs.ne.gov/licensure/Documents/ArtTherApplication.pdf

Nebraska Department of Health and Human Services. (2021). *Professional and occupational licensure credentialing review process*. Nebraska Secretary of State. Retrieved from www.nebraska.gov/rules-and-regs/regsearch/Rules/Health_and_Human_Services_System/Title-172/Chapter–004.pdf

Nebraska Legislature. (n.d.). *Law making in Nebraska*. Nebraska Legislature. Retrieved from https://nebraskalegislature.gov/about/lawmaking.php

Nebraska Legislature. (2024, March 12). *LB 605—change provisions of the mental health practice act to include protections and requirements for certified art therapy*. Nebraska

Legislature. Retrieved from https://nebraskalegislature.gov/bills/view_bill.php?DocumentID=49777

Putnam, R. D. (1994). Social capital and public affairs. *Bulletin of the American Academy of Arts and Sciences, 47*(8), 5–19. https://doi.org/10.2307/3824796

State of Nebraska. (2022). *Mental health practice act.* Department of Health and Human Services of Nebraska. Retrieved from https://dhhs.ne.gov/licensure/Documents/MentalHealthPracticeAct.pdf

van Rooijen, M. (2017, October 20). *Extrapreneurship is the future of entrepreneurship.* Retrieved from www.huffingtonpost.co.uk/professor-maurits-van-rooijen/extrapreneurship-is-the-f_b_12554610.html

*Chapter* **9**

# Academic Program Development as Social Entrepreneurship

*Jennifer Marie DeLucia*

Developing a new graduate program in art therapy was an opportunity I did not imagine I would have in my career. It was no coincidence that it materialized during a time when I was recognizing the need to bring more of my art therapist identity into my work at the University. Skills, experience, and relationships I developed over 15 years of professional practice in the field of art therapy uniquely prepared me for the challenge. Before joining the faculty at Syracuse University, I had developed an art therapy program at a community-based nonprofit, managed a successful private practice, established a local chapter of a national membership organization, and led a national community of practice that brought together service providers across federal, state, and community-based organizations. Through these experiences, I established skills in building collaborative relationships and working with groups of key partners to cocreate and implement new and innovative ideas.

My work as an educator is informed by my community-based approach to art therapy, my belief in art making as a way of knowing, and my entrepreneurial spirit. My desire to create and innovate is driven by my passionate sense of responsibility to the profession and to serve communities. Working with students as they prepare to enter the field of art therapy is a responsibility and an opportunity to advance the future of the profession by preparing ethical practitioners who are competent in contemporary issues and capable of leveraging their training for personal and social change, community development, and public health.

As an artist, art therapist, educator, and leader, I integrate beauty and authenticity into my work; I seek congruence between words, actions, and nonverbal expressions; and I strive to navigate complex problems while working to remain true to these values and principles (George, 2003). The

DOI: 10.4324/9781032615776-10

harmonious expression of purpose, values, and genuineness within professional relationships and the application of skillful leadership and authentic communication to working toward a common purpose define beautiful leadership (Ladkin, 2008). Viewing my work as a leader and educator through this aesthetic lens enables me to remain open to new possibilities and solutions, providing the space for cocreation of knowledge.

My experiences with arts-based and participatory action research have helped me hone my skills in collaborative problem-solving and cocreation of knowledge by working alongside people with lived experience who are impacted by the solutions generated in our research. Similarly, as a leader, I value art making and my responses to art as ways to deepen my understanding of complex situations, illuminate new questions or problems, and help guide innovative solutions. In addition to infusing this art-making practice in my classroom and my department's culture, I maintain an active art practice where I examine my work as an art therapist, leader, educator, and researcher.

## THE NEW DEPARTMENT'S ORIGIN STORY

My career at Syracuse University began in 2015, when I joined the University's Institute for Veterans and Military Families (IVMF) as a Senior Director. This role was a departure from my clinical and community-based work in the field of art therapy; however, I was eager to support the IVMF's initiative to improve service delivery for veterans and military-connected individuals across the nation. Working with federal, state, and community-based organizations, I developed a national community of practice to support the operation and continued performance improvement of more than a dozen coordinated care networks serving veterans and military-connected individuals.

Walking by classrooms en route to my office, I often imagined the prospect of someday teaching a graduate-level art therapy course at Syracuse University. Occasionally, a student would find my biography when searching for information about art therapy and contact me with questions about the field. I once teamed up with an undergraduate student at the University who was interested in seeing art therapy in action. We volunteered at a local nonprofit to give them experience and exposure to the field as they were considering a career in art therapy.

After working with the IVMF for a couple years, I became interested in how I could integrate more of my art therapist skills and identity into my work. A new building was being constructed that would include a veterans' art gallery. I saw this as an opportunity to propose how the gallery space could be used as a place for community connection and public education, drawing from my interest and background with using exhibitions in my art therapy practice.

Fast forward to the Annual Veterans Ball in April 2018. I had been circulating a gallery proposal and working with the Executive Director of the Office of Veteran and Military Affairs (OVMA) on campus to promote the concept. During the dinner, one of the student veterans asked the dean of the University's College of Visual and Performing Arts (VPA) about an art therapy program at the University. The dean responded that in fact an art therapy program was included in the College's strategic plan. In that moment, the Executive Director of the OVMA mentioned my recent proposal and offered to make an introduction. Subsequently, I received an email with an opportunity to meet with the dean and VPA College leadership. I knew this was a special opportunity. I prepared a proposal that provided a brief outline of the academic landscape of the field, along with a few models for a new art therapy program at the University.

In November 2018, I transitioned from my role at IVMF to the role of Director of Creative Arts Therapy in VPA. I was hired by the College to conduct a full feasibility study with the anticipation that the study would be successful and that I would move forward and lead in the development of a new graduate degree program. This transition enabled me to bridge my knowledge of community-based work and nonprofit leadership with my background in art therapy and experience in academia. The opportunity to research, propose, and ultimately develop a new graduate degree and academic department aligned with my interests in entrepreneurship and program development. On a personal level, the prospect of developing a new graduate program was exciting and terrifying. In some regards, I felt that everything I had tackled in my career up to this point had uniquely prepared me for the challenge. In other ways, it felt like an enormous undertaking, and I questioned if I was qualified. I have a high level of regard for the role the educators play in preparing students to enter the field. It is a great responsibility and privilege to serve the field in the capacity of an educator.

In December 2018, I initiated a feasibility study that explored the potential for low-residency graduate programming in art, music, and drama therapy. The second phase of the feasibility study was a more in-depth analysis of the potential for a new low-residency graduate program in art therapy specifically. Results from the research I conducted, involving interviews with program directors and American Art Therapy Association leadership, as well as analysis of program data collected from the Integrated Postsecondary Education Data System (IPEDS), were later validated by an external research firm. During this time, I chaired the campus Creative Arts Therapy Working Group, an advisory group comprised of members from across campus, including the IVMF, School of Education, Falk College of Sport and Human Dynamics, and VPA.

Our intent to create an online degree was socially oriented. We were responding to a need to increase access to art therapy training programs by reducing barriers some students may experience with traditional residential programs. Like most social entrepreneurial initiatives, we had to find a balance between addressing a social need and ensuring financial viability. This is particularly important in intrapreneurship, when change and innovation occur within an organization and the needs and goals of the broader institution need to be addressed. The results of our feasibility studies addressed the issue of sustainability, projecting that the investment made by the institution would result in a sustainable program.

In 2019, the program proposal received preapproval from the provost's office to move a full curriculum proposal forward through the University Curriculum Committee and Senate review process. The University Curriculum Committee and the Faculty Senate approved the full proposal in December 2019. Following the full university approval, the application was reviewed and approved by the New York State Department of Education in July 2020. This was a significant and celebrated milestone. The proposal went through all levels of approval uncontested and seamlessly. The COVID-19 pandemic that hit in March 2020 did not slow us down. As I was eager to move forward with developing courses, I had compressed the timeline for conducting a search and we filled a full-time faculty position by February 2020, just one month before all hiring actions were paused. At the time we launched in Fall 2021, the new graduate program was the fifth online art therapy degree program. In our initial year, we met our enrollment target, despite the potential challenges posed by the pandemic.

## PROGRAM DEVELOPMENT FRAMEWORK

The success of the program proposal can be attributed to the thoroughness of the research that went into the proposal, validation of the demand by an external research firm, and collaboration and support from leadership and partners across campus. This section of the chapter will provide a more detailed description of the research conducted to support the program proposal as well as provide an overview of the program model and curriculum development process.

### Field Research

The feasibility study was based on the present needs of the field and market demand. To better understand the current academic landscape in art therapy, I spoke with several art therapy program directors and faculty nationwide, as well the American Art Therapy Association president, communications and policy coordinator, and the Chair of the Assembly of Chapters. These conversations helped me to understand the potential demand for a new low-residency art therapy program, as well as current trends and issues in the field related to art therapy program accreditation and state licensure. I also reviewed online data on graduate art therapy programs, including accreditation status, completion rates, and areas of specialization. At that time, there were 39 graduate programs in art therapy in the United States. Of these 39 institutions, four offered an online or low-residency graduate program in art therapy. I learned that many programs offered part-time options or were moving toward evening classes to accommodate the needs of post-traditional or working students. Program directors also provided input and feedback on building cross-disciplinary collaborations, seeking accreditation, and building residency requirements to reduce barriers for post-traditional and international student participation.

Post-traditional learners are students who frequently must balance life, work, and their education. Many people I spoke with identified an increase in learners seeking this balance. Post-traditional learners are often already in the workforce and are earners for themselves or their families. They may also be parents, caregivers, or military-connected, either as a family member of an active-duty service member or veteran, or as a current or former service member (Soares et al., 2017). Often post-traditional students meet many or all of these characteristics. Low-residency programs offer flexibility to students seeking opportunities to further their education while maintaining these personal and professional commitments, in turn increasing accessibility and promoting diversity in the student body.

My goal was to design the program with current and future educational needs in mind. This required careful consideration of program accreditation options. In response to the complicated landscape of professional licensure in art therapy, some programs were modeled to meet the counseling accreditation requirements, while others aligned with the art therapy accreditation requirements. During the initial field research and market analysis, conversations with program directors and leaders helped me understand how other programs were navigating this decision. Ultimately, we decided that aligning with art therapy accreditation requirements was the right decision for our program, and one that I believe aligned with the future of the profession, as many states were advocating and lobbying for art therapy licenses—ultimately over time reducing (with the goal of eliminating) the need for art therapists to pursue counseling licenses.

## Market Analysis

In July 2019, an external research firm completed a formal market analysis to satisfy the University's requirement that new program proposals undergo formal evaluation to determine market viability. I also conducted my own market analysis as part of the program proposal. My initial analysis covered a rationale for the new program, a detailed overview of the profession, curriculum competency requirements, graduate program admission requirements, demand for a low-residency program with comparison of completion rates at competitor institutions, overview of cost competitiveness, job outlook for graduates, and the projected enrollment and revenue assumptions provided by VPA's senior director of Budget, Operations and Strategic Initiatives. The proposal also discussed how the program fits within the college's and University's missions and visions.

I provided a copy of my analysis to the hired consultants conducting the analysis. This facilitated a successful outcome, as the firm was not familiar with the field of art therapy and the study provided background information needed to inform their approach. Through a combination of qualitative interviews with administrators of comparable programs, quantitative data analytics, and secondary research, the firm assessed the market demand for a low-residency master-level art therapy program. The study affirmed my research findings and served as an important benchmark for the proposal to pass through the various levels of approval at the University. It was determined that there was a viable market for a new low-residency art therapy program.

## College Leadership

VPA's dean, the associate dean of Academic Affairs, the associate dean of Graduate Studies, Research and Internationalization, and the senior director of Budget, Operations, and Strategic Initiatives provided support and access to the resources and relationships necessary for the proposal to be successful. During the initial year, when I was independently working on the feasibility study and program proposal, I provided brief reports to leadership by email or through in-person meetings to keep them informed of the progress. I was not familiar with many of the University's processes and academic culture, and the leadership team helped to fill that knowledge gap. Their investment, assistance, and mentorship were crucial to the success of the initiative—and also acted as an anchor for me in the process.

## Cross-Disciplinary Advisory Team

Early in the development process, the dean convened a group of staff and faculty from across campus to serve in an advisory capacity. He provided the initial charge for the group with me serving as the Chair. The Creative Arts Therapy Graduate Program Working Group was comprised of members from Syracuse University's IVMF, School of Education, David B. Falk College of Sport and Human Dynamics, and several programs across VPA. In an advisory capacity, the working group provided feedback on proposal documents and helped to ensure the success of the proposal by promoting buy-in and support across related areas of the University. I convened the group in person at several key points in the process and members also made themselves available to review documents and provide feedback by email as necessary.

## Campus Partnerships

To further promote opportunities for collaboration, I facilitated partnerships with colleagues from the School of Education's Clinical Mental Health Counseling and Falk College's Department of Marriage and Family Therapy. Collectively, we were interested in cross-disciplinary collaboration on course offerings for students, providing opportunities for students to participate in interdisciplinary learning. Through these partnerships, we added three required art therapy courses that can be taught by faculty in related professions. All art therapy students take at least one course with marriage and family therapy faculty and two courses with counseling faculty. There are also other opportunities for students to take elective courses in these areas.

# SYRACUSE UNIVERSITY'S MODEL

The decision to develop a low-residency graduate training program in art therapy was in response to the need for accessible learning opportunities. The program was designed to meet the needs of post-traditional students and students who were otherwise not able to relocate for graduate school. While the online program may not address concerns about tuition costs, it does address financial barriers in other ways. Online education reduces costs associated with relocating to attend the program, transportation (e.g., gas, tolls, parking), and childcare. The program schedule is modeled in a way that enables students to work full-time and balance caregiving responsibilities. All courses are offered in the evenings and most courses are a blend of synchronous and asynchronous sessions. Most textbooks are offered online through the University library, bringing additional cost savings to students who use the available eBooks. We decided that a low-residency model with two required in-person residencies would support the delivery of the curriculum and provide maximum flexibility to prospective students.

The learning objectives of the program parallel those of traditional on-campus programs and emphasize community and cohort development. The program follows a cohort model; students are admitted in the fall and progress through the three-year program together as a group. In the fall of the first year and the fall of the second year, the cohort gathers for an in-person residency on Syracuse University's main campus. The year one residency provides students an opportunity to orient to the program objectives, online tools, and to begin to develop a cohesive and supportive learning community among cohort members and faculty. In year two, students return for a second residency. This second residency provides an opportunity for students to meet with faculty to complete the required student performance review and clinical simulations.

During each residency, students begin their fall course work in person and are oriented to the online approach for completing the remainder of their coursework online. Online instruction includes live, synchronous sessions that continue to build open communication and group cohesion. Asynchronous content, which includes prerecorded lectures and discussion boards, reinforces a student-centered approach where students can flexibly maintain engagement with the community and material during times convenient for their schedules. Asynchronous activities also help to reinforce the sense of community among cohort members by providing students the opportunity to share thoughts and respond to assignments and reflections.

Relationships between faculty and students are developed and supported through various opportunities including residency, synchronous sessions, and asynchronous content. Synchronous sessions provide opportunities for students to engage with faculty in real-time and offer the same anchor and regular touchpoint that students receive in traditional on-campus programs. Asynchronous content and assignments are developed in a way that promotes collaboration and communication among cohort members. Faculties are also available through regular and flexible remote office hours, where they connect with students through live video or phone calls.

The quality of instructor feedback in each course parallels the high standards held in traditional programs, while the quantity of feedback meets and, in many cases, exceeds traditional programs. Faculty use consistent, thoughtful feedback to promote engagement, coach students to successful completion of the program, and challenge students to achieve at their highest potential. Upon completion of the program, students are prepared to be competent and ethical practitioners, qualified for professional practice, licensure, and national certification. Program learning objectives and clinical preparation align with the highest national standards for art therapists practicing in the United States.

## Creating a Community of Learners

Reflexive learning is at the center of our approach to creating a collaborative environment where students and faculty alike contribute to the learning community. Reflexive learning views students as cocreators of knowledge, promoting exchanges between students and instructors and between students and students (Fataar & Norodien-Fataar, 2021). Reflexivity also involves an awareness and examination of how factors like power dynamics and social context influence how knowledge is constructed (Ryan & Walsh, 2018). Synchronous and asynchronous activities in each course provide a range of opportunities for students to develop self-awareness, critical thinking skills, and empathy, by asking critical questions like, "How did my experiences shape my perspective?" Using the range of tools available, online learning environments can engage multiple types of learners through a blend of live and asynchronous activities, providing opportunities for diverse types of learners to be successful. Students have opportunities to engage through written and artistic reflection in one-to-one exchanges with the professor in their weekly journal and with their peers on the discussion board. In live sessions, students engage verbally with the class as a whole and with smaller breakout groups. Reflexivity promotes culturally responsive teaching through a supportive and collaborative learning environment that acknowledges and affirms students' cultural identities and lived experiences. As cocreators of knowledge, students actively contribute to their community of learners.

## Curriculum Development

Curriculum development involved creating initial syllabi for all courses that would be offered in the program. The syllabi were a required component of the program proposal for the University's and the New York Department of Education's approval. The courses were designed to meet articulated student learning outcomes and required content areas outlined by the Accreditation Council for Art Therapy Education (ACATE). Once the course objectives and content areas were mapped onto each course, assignments, readings, and activities for each week were developed. To accomplish this task in the compressed time allocated, I brought in a consultant to help with development. In addition to aligning with ACATE requirements, we focused on infusing contemporary practice trends and issues into the curriculum. We focused on key areas, including integrating a focus on social and cultural diversity into each course by incorporating literature and content that represented multiple perspectives and experiences. Critical analysis of stereotypes, biases, and inequalities was also infused in the curriculum and reinforced at multiple points throughout.

## Recruiting and Hiring Faculty

Once the program was approved, I received permission to hire a full-time professor of practice to help develop the first-year courses. We had one year to work together on program development before the official launch with our inaugural cohort. I prioritized hiring faculty who had experience in online learning as either a learner or an instructor; ideal candidates had experience with both. It was also important to recruit team members who were enthusiastic about contributing to the development of a new program. The nature of the role required faculty who were collaborative by nature, highly organized, and comfortable with some degree of uncertainty. Our second faculty hire was a tenure-track position that started with the program in August 2021, as the program launched. The two faculty positions were structured around particular skill sets that would align with the courses each faculty member would be responsible for developing. The initial hire was focused on foundational courses and supporting development of the program's internship procedures and practices. The second hire was focused on advanced courses in the program and the program's thesis and culminating project requirements. As co-collaborators on the next phase of development, we initially met as a department weekly to promote a culture of collaboration and cross-sharing of ideas.

## Course Development Process

Methods for building online courses vary among institutions depending on the resources available. Syracuse University's Center for Online and Digital Learning (CODL) is a university-wide resource available to programs developing new online courses. CODL uses instructional design theories, prescriptive models, and research to leverage the full spectrum of learning possible through technology-enhanced environments (Syracuse University, n.d.). An instructional designer works with a faculty member to guide them through the design and production process, provides ideas for creating engaging and interactive lessons, and works with the video production team to execute course design (Syracuse University Center for Online and Digital Learning, n.d.).

Course preparation and design in online learning poses new challenges for many faculty, like the requirement that they prepare (and upload) course materials well in advance of launching the course (Hillman et al., 2021). In the initial phase of course development, the professor creates an outline of the course that includes content, activities, and learning objectives for each week. The professor then works with the instructional designer to delineate what portions of the content will be delivered in synchronous sessions and what will be covered in asynchronous sessions. The timeframe for developing a course from start to finish can range from six to ten months, depending on the amount of time the faculty member can devote to course development. VPA's investment of resources to retain two full-time faculty to devote one full academic year to develop the first six art therapy courses was necessary to ensure the materials were developed and finalized in time for the program launch.

Students vary in the ways they learn best. Some are visual learners and benefit from visual aids to illustrate material, others learn better through auditory methods like lectures or discussions, and some are more oriented around kinetic learning through hands-on activities and interactive experiences (Hillman et al., 2021). The range of tools available to faculty teaching online courses supports a diverse approach that engages students in multiple methods of learning. The designers at CODL helped to ensure the University's standards for universal design were met by attending to issues of accessibility throughout the course development process. Designers also helped faculty to consider the most engaging and memorable way to deliver the content, including the use of animation, graphics, and illustrations that can be embedded in the recorded sessions.

Courses developed for our art therapy program include interactive recorded lectures—some of which feature demonstrations or role play—and asynchronous activities and experiential learning that support engagement with the material through art making, online discussions, and personal reflective journaling. Each course includes synchronous sessions and asynchronous components every week. Discussion boards, email, weblog interactions, and voice conversations via telephone, Skype, and Adobe Connect were all used to provide additional flexible interaction with faculty and among students. Art making is also a central feature in both synchronous and asynchronous sessions. Students have access to a studio for art making during the program's two required residencies and are provided with a range of opportunities during the online portions of the program to engage with the curriculum through personal art making and art-making interactions among cohort members.

## MAINTAINING A CULTURE OF COLLABORATION

At the same time our new program was approved, our new Department of Creative Arts Therapies was also established within VPA. Creative arts therapies include the regulated professions of art therapy, dance/movement therapy, music therapy, and drama therapy. The department plans to explore the potential for low-residency training programs in some of these areas.

As a department chair, I have worked to foster and maintain a collaborative environment that promotes cocreation and values the contribution of diverse ideas and perspectives. Collaboration is a core value I promote in our department, one I seeded early on when developing the new academic unit and program in art therapy. This is evidenced by our department's strong relationships with collaborative partners across campus.

All department faculty and staff have worked together on a collaborative painting (see Figure 9.1) during in-person department meetings held throughout the year. I initiated this collaborative and ongoing art process to invite new faculty into the development of our new department and art therapy program. Each faculty and staff member contributes to areas of program development (including research, internship, and the program's art gallery) that align with their strengths and interests. Engaging in art making as a group has become a ritual for coming together, and the collaborative surface on the canvas parallels the environment of cocreation we strive to maintain in the department.

## CONCLUSION

Educational literature has identified that in-person learning was "ripe for radical transformation" and that the rapid transition to online modalities during the COVID-19 pandemic highlighted the issues with didactic styles of teaching (Kalantzis & Cope, 2012, as cited in Fataar & Norodien-Fataar, 2021, p. 161). Leveraging the capacity of technology for multimodal learning supports a level of intellectual engagement that prepares students as "knowledge producers for critical citizenship" (Fataar & Norodien-Fataar, 2021, p. 163). Technology is interwoven into our personal, social, and educational lives; critical engagement with technology in education represents a contemporary approach in response to the current needs and interests of students (Fataar & Norodien-Fataar, 2021).

The accessibility promoted by low-residency programs can help to seed art therapy in new regions across the country as well as internationally. We have seen this to slowly develop in Syracuse, NY, as small nonprofit

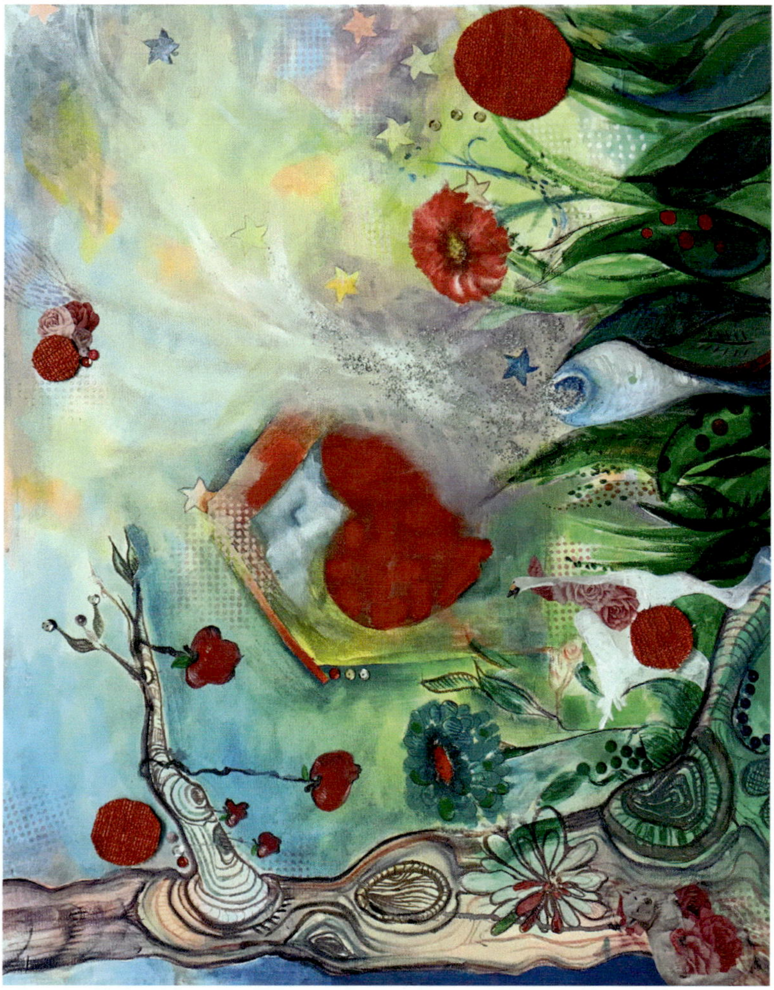

***Figure 9.1*** *Cocreation: Building Together.*

*Note.* Collaborative mix-media painting with tree, heart, flowers, and foliage completed by Department of Creative Arts Therapy faculty and staff, Jennifer Marie DeLucia, Emily Goldstein Nolan, Rochele Royster, and Emma Rathe, on a 24" x 36" stretched canvas.

organizations reach out to the department to host art therapy interns and consider how they might sustain art therapy programs within their settings. Low-residency programs also promote access to post-traditional students by reducing barriers associated with relocating. More institutions are embracing this approach to program delivery, evidenced by the significant post-pandemic growth in online programs.

At the time I am writing this, we are preparing to graduate our first cohort of students—we are eager to witness the contributions this group of trailblazers will make in their communities and the field of art therapy. We are also eager to continue to grow our community of learners each year as we expand our reach geographically and help to promote access to art therapy education.

## REFERENCES

Fataar, A., & Norodien-Fataar, N. (2021). Towards an e-learning ecologies approach to pedagogy in a post-COVID world. *Journal of Education, 84*, 155–168.

George, B. (2003). *Authentic leadership: Rediscovering the secrets to creating lasting value.* Jossey-Bass.

Hillman, D., Schudy, R., & Temkin, A. (2021). *Best practices for administering online programs.* Routledge.

Kalantzis, M., & Cope, B. (2012). New learning: A charter for change in education. *Critical Studies in Education, 53*(1), 83–94.

Ladkin, D. (2008). Leading beautifully: How mastery, congruence and purpose create the aesthetic of embodied leadership practice. *Leadership Quarterly, 19*(1), 31–41.

Ryan, A., & Walsh, T. (2018). Reflexivity and critical pedagogy. In A. Ryan, T. Walsh, & P. Mayo (Eds.), *Reflexive and critical pedagogy* (pp. 1–14). Brill.

Soares, L., Gagliardi, J. S., & Nellum, C. J. (2017). *The post-traditional leaners manifesto revisited: Aligning postsecondary education with real like for adult student success.* American Council on Education. Retrieved April 18, 2024, from www.acenet.edu/Documents/The-Post-Traditional-Learners-Manifesto-Revisited.pdf

Syracuse University. (n.d.). *Center for online and digital learning.* Retrieved April 18, 2024, from https://professionalstudies.syracuse.edu/about/office-directory/center-for-online-and-digital-learning/

Syracuse University Center for Online and Digital Learning. (n.d.). *Course building guidebook* [Unpublished document]. Center for Online and Digital Learning, Syracuse University.

*Chapter* **10**

# The Ripple Effect of Entrepreneurship

## Increasing Impact Through Evolution

*Emery Hurst Mikel*

### INTRODUCTION

I have never really followed a predictable path in life and have always aimed to do things that felt engaging and meaningful. When I have to make a choice about which direction to go, I take a moment to think; I strive to say yes more often than not, sometimes even surprising myself. Most of the paths I have traveled have led to greater wisdom and insight into myself and the world. This chapter is focused on the stage of my journey that begins with my first step into the world of social entrepreneurship as a traveling art therapist and continues to the moment I formed my own group practice, Water & Stone, a Creative Arts Therapy PLLC. This stage of my adventure illustrates how becoming a social entrepreneur can start with an idea that transforms over time into something with a potential impact rarely fathomed when that first thought or question initially surfaces.

I have been self-employed since 2008. I am passionate about bringing art therapy into the community in innovative and accessible ways and supporting therapists in finding their unique paths, no matter how big or small their dream is. Currently, I run two companies in New York City—a group practice and a business supporting therapists—and teach as adjunct faculty in graduate programs. I had ideas and dreams during graduate school, but never could have envisioned the remarkable reality that unfolded over the years. I hope by sharing my story, you can find some inspiration, encouragement, and confidence to move forward in whatever direction feels right for you.

DOI: 10.4324/9781032615776-11

## THE STORY

### The Ebb and Flow of My Journey

During high school in the 1990s, Ms. Gloria Dossett saw something in me that helped me transform from shy student to passionate leader over my four years acting and directing in The Madeira School theater department. This passion continued to evolve at Carnegie Mellon University where I could deeply immerse myself in the exploration of what it takes to guide a team of artistic professionals toward a cohesive goal—a performance that holds the power to deeply connect with and speak to each member of the audience. How amazing to create an entire world and experience for those watching, and hopefully make an impact emotionally and psychologically!

Several years after graduating with my BFA in Drama with a concentration in directing, this love of making an impact grew into a desire to help people create lifelong changes and better understand themselves. I explored various psychological pursuits, but when my mother found art therapy, I was all in! A unique program at Naropa University aligned with the sense I had of how I saw community and relationships in the world, so off to Colorado I went for three years to get my master's degree in Transpersonal Counseling Psychology and Art Therapy. I found a deeper connection than I ever could have anticipated and was excited to explore new options for working with people upon my return to Washington D.C. Luckily, a horrendous job right out of graduate school led to a conversation with my ATR supervisor in 2007 that inspired the vision of becoming a traveling art therapist to come to light, offering group therapy to older adults who would not otherwise be able to access such services.

I researched business topics, created initial paperwork, and went through a year of trial and error as my plan came into focus. Once I developed a reliable system and had 20 locations a month to visit, I welcomed interns from George Washington University. Two years with interns taught me so much before the time came to move out of state to Long Island, N.Y., in 2010. I devised a way to transfer my traveling art therapy business to two other art therapists in the hopes it would help them jumpstart their own work and my clients would still have art therapy.

Long Island brought new challenges and possibilities as I rebuilt a similar program to D.C. while recognizing the many ways I needed to adapt or innovate. I learned a lot about flexibility before moving to Brooklyn in 2013 when I began teaching in graduate art therapy programs and finding ways to expand the types of services I offered. In 2015, I founded Water & Stone, a Creative Arts Therapy PLLC and other therapists began asking "how do you run a private practice?" I recognized the limitations of working alone and researched how to hire independent contractors. Over the next few years, my group practice grew to include twelve creative arts therapists and three offices in Manhattan and Brooklyn. Things were thriving, but I was about to have to pivot again.

With 2020, came COVID-19 and the world shut down. I closed all our offices, spoke to my therapists, and we shifted to a totally virtual existence. We adapted and stabilized in a new world. I was getting so many requests from therapists asking for help starting private practices that I was inspired to start a second small business, Firefly & Phoenix LLC, in 2021. Water & Stone supports the community and therapy clients, while Firefly & Phoenix focuses on helping professionals develop the work they dream of doing in their communities. The evolution of Firefly & Phoenix is for another time, but it is amazing to feel everything came full circle from my supervisor helping me find my passion to my helping other therapists find theirs.

## THE ORIGINAL INSPIRATION

Inspiration and an adventure I had not anticipated were borne out of having a horrible job and knowing something had to change. I was living in Maryland at the time and in supervision for my registered art therapist credential with Carol T. Cox. Carol was paramount in helping me explore what it was I truly wanted to do. I had always been passionate about working with older adults with dementia. However, they could not easily access services like art therapy. Beyond that, the facilities they lived in often saw the benefits of art therapy but did not have the budget to hire a full-time art therapist. My vision turned into a quest to develop a program for older adults living in facilities that made art therapy accessible and the program sustainable.

Once I had the vision in mind, the hurdles that appeared became a creative puzzle. Who can afford this, at what price? Where can I work? What does accessible mean for this population? How do I make this sustainable for me and affordable for the facility? How can I create community for my clients? What are the first steps in this bigger vision?

The exciting and daunting path that began to reveal itself focused on building a traveling art therapy practice that could reach multiple facilities serving older adults within a certain geographic radius. I could work at multiple sites each week, bring supplies with me, and run groups to keep costs down. My hope was that clients would benefit from the social nature of the group while engaging in creativity to promote a better quality of life. It was exciting to have a clear vision!

## THE EVOLUTION

Once I had the focus, I dove into researching marketing, paperwork, and taxes, and tackled many other unknowns. I developed a marketing packet that included my information as well as a photo of a piece of art I had created with a group. I looked online and in books for what it meant to be an independent contractor. I also tried to figure out pricing. I will say I got that one totally wrong at first, but learned quickly!

The most challenging moment was deciding when I knew enough to actually run a group. Trusting that pivotal point and diving into a more trial-and-error stage was terrifying. Luckily, my first group went well with the clients and facility. However, I was undercharging ($50/hour.) and overpromising ("We'll make a quilt!"), so I had to quickly adjust expectations and boundaries. The most incredible realization from those first jobs was understanding that it was okay to learn as things unfolded over time.

An important note: the risks I was taking focused on the business side of things. I had worked with this population in multiple settings over several years, so I was very comfortable running the groups. It was important to me, personally and ethically, to keep the therapy work I was doing within my areas of expertise while taking so many new steps into being an entrepreneur.

For three years, I built up my traveling art therapy clientele to include community centers, retirement homes, and day programs. Interns joined me from George Washington University with the enthusiastic support of Lisa Garlock, the internship coordinator at the time. I learned an immense amount and embraced the idea of healthy risk taking. It was a balance of doing my due diligence to learn what I did not know and letting trial and error be a part of my approach. I valued questions and got excited about learning new ways of doing things. I also practiced embracing failure and seeing it as a helpful tool. Most importantly, I sought out support from mentors or friends to help keep me engaged and to embrace a mindset of possibility.

## NEW YORK

In 2010, I planned to move to New York. Lisa Garlock gave me the idea of selling my business, and I advertised for and found two therapists willing to shadow me for a month and each would take over half my clientele. The experience was illuminating for me. I loved sharing what I had done and the systems I had created. To know that my clients would continue to have groups and two therapists got a jump start on this kind of work was exhilarating.

New challenges awaited me in New York and after recreating some of my traveling work on Long Island, I realized I would need to adapt more than I anticipated to my new environment. I spent two years navigating new facilities and New York's licensing process. It was challenging and felt like I was on pause. Then, with a license in hand, I moved to Brooklyn and everything began to change.

I gave up my car and while traveling to run groups throughout Brooklyn and Manhattan was exciting, it was also exhausting! Running around the city, taking subways and buses was good for some things, but was not sustainable, so I shifted gears. I found an office in Dumbo where I could have a home base. I limited the traveling and started welcoming clients dealing with grief and loss into my office. My vision grew and I started developing variety in my work: traveling to sites, seeing individuals, and running occasional workshops for therapists.

## WATER & STONE

As I hit a limit with my own time and energy, I dreamed of having a wider impact. Friends and colleagues had been asking how I was able to do all of this, and I realized there were ways I could support people in the community that went beyond just me. It was scary, but it was time for another leap.

I created Water & Stone, a Creative Arts Therapy PLLC, in 2015 to encompass what I hoped would eventually be a small group practice. Water & Stone expanded over the next couple of years to include 12 creative arts therapists with three offices in Brooklyn and Manhattan. All worked independently as contractors, but I took care of the business side of things. They could do private practice in their way and reach clients they felt passionate about working with. I saw a few of my own clients, ran the businesses, and started running more workshops and offering continuing education hours for therapists. We were reaching so many people. It was a dream come true.

Then 2020 and the COVID-19 pandemic happened, and once again, I had to help my company and vision evolve. We pivoted to virtual work, I let the offices go, and for a while Water & Stone just held steady. We had a couple of challenging years in the aftermath of the pandemic and are now rebuilding and finding new ways, once again, to meet the needs of the community. Sometimes it is tiring, but overall, it is awe-inspiring that we get to do this work in this way.

## BEYOND WATER & STONE

While Water & Stone held steady, another opportunity presented itself. Many therapists were interested in private practice post-pandemic, so

I developed new programs to support others in finding their visions and realizing their dreams. People were interested in the support and the programs grew until what I was offering could no longer fit under the Water & Stone umbrella. For clarity, both for the therapists and myself, I founded a new company, Firefly & Phoenix LLC, in 2023. That is a story for another book, but suffice it to say, the evolution of my original vision has taken me in directions I never expected to go. The ways I hope to impact the world continue to grow and change every year.

## IMPORTANT TOPICS AND THOUGHTS

### Vision and Innovation

The Traveling Vision

In 2008, my leap into social entrepreneurship came from a dream of bringing weekly art therapy to groups of older adults and people who could not easily access services, by traveling to multiple facilities and organizations while working within common budgetary constraints of the systems in which these populations existed. The secondary goal was to create community while doing so.

*Innovating for the Initial Vision*

After the idea came the planning. I researched and read books on business skills, looked through posts online about private practice, and scoured the internet for examples or stories of what people had done before. I could not find much that was helpful or published specifically about art therapy, so I had to be creative and innovative.

From the information I found, as well as a good amount of trial and error, I created a marketing packet, paperwork (invoice, contract, W-9), a short script for the first phone contact, and explored pricing. There was a balance and flow between searching for new information, learning how to approach various tasks, and taking a step forward by putting what I learned into action.

As the nuts and bolts came together, I was also focused on developing the creative side, figuring out the best ways to bring art therapy to the groups at their facilities. I devised an organizational system of containers to hold various materials, so I could easily transport what was needed for that day's sessions. I also planned out a series of objectives and topics that involved cycling through different types of materials, so I could better meet the needs of the people I was working with. I was determined to bring a variety of materials, create tactile experiences, and inspire each person's inner artist.

### The Water & Stone Vision

I was inspired to build community and support more clients gaining access to creative arts therapy, by starting a group practice focused on contemplative psychotherapy and creative arts therapy.

#### *Innovations for Water & Stone*

Everything I created for Water & Stone developed from what I had made when traveling as an art therapist. It was amazing to let ideas, paperwork, and how I described the work to the community evolve and find new purposes. I developed a few new systems and stayed open to the unknown as we started.

Some of the developments I focused my energy on included creating supervision groups to support others and build community, reworking paperwork, making sure the new therapists had everything they needed, and revamping my approach to marketing with a website and information encompassing creative arts therapy rather than just art therapy and myself. One of the hardest transitions was becoming the voice of a group practice and wanting everyone to feel represented. There was a lot of discussion and input from those who joined me and I made it a point to ask for help, guidance, and ideas to keep myself from operating in a bubble of my own thoughts. Developing these new ways of connecting my vision and our mission with the community was a bit scary at first, but also brought an inspiring new level of creativity and possibility to what I had started.

## MANAGING RISK

### Healthy Risk Taking

One thing I learned is how important it is to embrace the idea that what we think of as failing is actually a wonderful and important way of learning and growing as an entrepreneur. So many things will not go as planned the first time. Often because we are trying something that has not been done or we are adapting to a new situation. Embrace these moments and practice intentionally taking risks without expecting perfection. What would you do if it were okay to fail the first time and you knew you would have more chances to adjust and try again?

## Aim for Good Enough and Competent

Wisdom and expertise will develop over time, but we do not start out there. We have to have experiences to gain that level of understanding for any topic or endeavor. On the other end of the spectrum is someone who is uninformed and foolish. This shows up when we dive into something without any preparation or do not seek out a base level understanding of what we are stepping into. The goal is to find the middle ground, where we are good enough to start and competent enough to be informed as we take our first steps in a direction. For example, before starting Water & Stone, I researched different business structures, redid paperwork, and explored organizations in the area with whom I might connect. At that point, I was ready to make contact and take my first steps.

## Risks I Took

When I finally jumped into my first group as a traveling art therapist in 2008, I thought most things went well. Then the activity director asked for a W-9 and an invoice. I smiled and said I would get those to her. I had no clue what a W-9 was at that point and did not know how to make an invoice. I did some Googling when I got home and learned a lot in the process! I also realized, within a few weeks, that I was undercharging for the group and I was losing money. I asked for a higher rate from new contacts while putting a plan in place with the first site to increase the amount over time.

### *Interns*

Taking on interns was challenging and there was a lot to figure out. It took time and energy, plus I had to explain myself in ways I usually did not have to. It felt risky. What if I did it wrong or could not answer a question? Of course, I occasionally messed something up, but I learned how to guide the interns and set up valuable experiences. The challenges became learning moments for both the interns and myself.

### *Saying No and Turning Down Clients*

At first, I tried to fill all requests from facilities or clients. It took a little while, and a lot of stress, to realize it was okay to say, "I don't know, but let me get back to you about that" or "I'm sorry, that's not something we offer." They either adapted or decided it did not fit. Either way I could move forward.

*Taking on Other Therapists as Independent Contractors*

I had to let go of control. All I could do was set up a supportive structure, good paperwork, and trust them to be good therapists while checking in now and then. Over time, I found we could work through most challenges that arose and by creating a group practice based on openness and trust, people felt safe coming to me when there were issues or if they had questions.

## CREATIVITY AND LEADERSHIP SKILLS

To me, creativity and leadership go hand in hand. To be a good leader, I have to see multiple perspectives and find creative solutions. People are diverse and unique, so both come into play as I navigate each new situation or challenge.

Leadership was first about the development of what I was offering the community and over time leadership evolved into how I presented myself, and the field of art therapy. As I mentored therapists and eventually hired people, leadership became about guiding, teaching, and supporting each person in becoming the best version of their unique selves.

Creativity is what made this entire journey possible. As an artist, and former theater director, I find myself using my creativity in marketing, managing people, developing new programs, and connecting with the community. Sometimes it is about designing flyers, social media posts, and creating examples of interventions. At other times, it is more about my directing side showing up in how I choose to listen to the therapists working with me and take their perspectives and experiences into account before guiding us toward the vision I am holding for the company. I think one of the most amazing ways creativity supports my work is the fun, out-of-the-box thinking I enjoy when developing a new workshop or program. Bringing something into the world that was not there and seeing how it both creates and transforms the community is inspiring. On a personal level, creating my own art is how I process and express myself. It brings new ideas into focus, visually shows me where I am or where I want to go next, and holds both the celebrations and the challenges I have faced.

I truly believe that creative arts therapists are in a unique position to develop programs, practices, and innovative means of meeting the needs of society. It is easier to learn business skills or hire someone to do that side of the work than it is to learn how to see multiple perspectives and think outside of the box.

## BUSINESS AND MANAGERIAL SKILLS

This is the hardest for many people! The business and managerial side of the work I do took practice and patience. I was fortunate to have amazing training in my undergraduate education as a theater director and stage manager. It helped hone a lot of the skills I still use when managing my companies and started me off on the right foot as I brought my programs to the community. Find a way to be more organized, practice setting aside time for tasks like marketing, and intersperse skills you are better at with ones that challenge you.

### Not Everyone Needs to Like You

Look for people who are curious and believe in what you have to offer. As you put ideas and possibilities out into the world, do not worry when someone does not want your services or is not interested in your vision. That is fine and you can then shift your focus elsewhere. It is not a personal affront and usually has nothing to do with you. It is just not a good fit at that moment.

### Burning Bridges

There is no telling what is going on in someone's life the moment you make contact or what current circumstances keep them from wanting to work with you. We also cannot see the future, so err on the side of professional understanding. I have had contacts change jobs and immediately reach out to explain why they could not hire me then but want to now. I also had a person collect my marketing materials for 6 months before remembering to follow up with a phone call. It is challenging, but unless I hear "No, we don't need what you are offering." I keep getting in touch. When I hear "no," I say thank you and I would love to hear from them if anything changes in the future.

### Face Fears Head-on

Anything you are nervous about or uncertain about, face head-on. If you worry, clients will cancel and not pay you, clarify your cancellation policy in the paperwork. If you are unclear about the site's parameters for when you run your program, call and ask all the questions you have. If you are not sure exactly what the people you hope to support need, ask them. The worst-case scenario is that you risk annoying or angering someone by your policy or questions. In that case, you have more information that can help you decide how long you want to continue the relationship.

### Listen

Listen to people when they speak. If someone feels heard and respected, even if you cannot meet all their needs, you have made a good connection and probably learned a few things. Especially on the marketing side, I see people speak and try to sell their services way too quickly. Be informative and then hear what the person is saying. As a therapist, I get to be a person and a professional, not a stereotypical salesman. I would rather build connections than sell my services. In the long term, there is a much greater benefit for all.

## MENTORSHIP AND COMMUNITY

### Find Your Community and Mentors

Don't do it alone! Often, social entrepreneurship means you are creating wonderful ways to serve others and meet the needs of the community. Having your own support system can make all the difference while following your path. I intentionally looked for different forms of support, so I would not feel isolated or get stuck in my head. At the start, I had mentors and friends I could bounce ideas off. Most of these people had no direct experience with anything like what I was doing, but they could listen and offer constructive feedback and compassion. That was invaluable. As things progressed, and I could afford it, I found professionals who could take on aspects of the work I struggled with or that I needed to take off my plate. Currently, I have an amazing virtual assistant who takes on many tasks and helps me determine what I do not need to do myself, so I can free up time for more important or creative endeavors.

### Mentor and Support Others

Mentor and teach people. It can be so inspiring! It can also keep you energized and compassionately humble. Explaining how I do things, and then supporting others to find their own way reminds me that I am thriving and that I started out with loads of questions and uncertainty. Whether I am working with interns, students, new therapists, or seasoned professionals, I love seeing others work through challenges to find their next steps and ultimately feel proud about what they are doing.

## SUSTAINABILITY

Keeping my vision, and the impact it could have on the community, in mind, has been pivotal to building something sustainable. It is important to let that vision grow or change. Sustainability does not mean you reach a certain point and nothing changes. To remain healthy as a person and a company, there is natural evolution. Embrace it! The alternative is holding too tight to a vision that no longer fits (or it is not time for yet) and stagnating. This leads to burnout. Here are some thoughts about what makes a dream or vision sustainable.

### Time Is a Weird Thing

It takes time to realize a dream and to make an impact on the world. That's okay! Enjoy what you are currently working on and the successes you have, no matter how big or small. At the same time, get excited about the hiccups and failures. I love hearing no, or coming away from a workshop thinking "Well, that did not go as planned." These are the opportunities to explore and find new ways to work. You do not know if that thing that went so badly actually gives you new insight or ideas that will pay off in amazing ways down the road. It takes time to have hindsight and to see what was actually helpful on your journey. Be wary of the need for immediate gratification and your initial self-judgments. Take the time to let things evolve. Trust yourself and your vision.

### Diversify Your Services

I offer a lot of different services to several communities. This keeps my work life interesting and lessens the impact when one aspect of my work is struggling. No one has to do as many different things as I do, but consider if there is a way for you to offer two or three different services. Or, would you like to work with people in the community as well as develop materials to support them in ways they can use on their own? Think through how to balance what you would like to do and how you can offer it in a couple of ways you enjoy.

### Flexibility and Adaptation

What happens when you are following the path you created and a new opportunity pops up? Does veering off the path you had planned to follow totally derail your dream or might it deepen your work in a way you had not anticipated? It is hard to know the right answer, so remaining flexible and open to changing course is important. If it does not feel like it aligns, great, say no. Just do not confuse unexpected with misaligned. There is no way to know what lies ahead or to see all the possibilities around us. Make one choice at a time and take healthy risks.

### Vision versus First Step

The vision of where you are going or what you want to do is your inspiration. At the same time, do not try to fully realize your vision on day one. Know the difference between where you are headed and what your next step is. Your vision will inspire you, your steps will get you there. If you are feeling overwhelmed or stuck, like you cannot move forward, often the focus is on something too far in the future, as opposed to your next few steps. Trust yourself and your process.

### Get Support

This is worth saying over and over. Find people to be a part of your dream and do not try to do it alone. First, it might be supportive friends who you can talk to when you are stuck or stressed out about something. Next you might find a peer support group of like-minded individuals. It is okay to find free or reasonably priced resources first and then, once you can afford it, look for people to take things off your plate (accounting, social media, creating a newsletter, scheduling, etc.). I have had friends and colleagues step into various roles over time and now have a wonderful virtual assistant. It took time to find the right people, but the difference it makes is immeasurably beneficial to my company and myself.

## CURRENT AND FUTURE VISIONS FOR MY JOURNEY AS A SOCIAL ENTREPRENEUR

Water & Stone went through some challenges across 2020–2022 and it is taking time to rebuild and envision the new opportunities for my group practice. The wonderful thing that came out of these challenges was the chance to focus on supporting other therapists and developing that side of my work in the creative arts therapy community. In 2023, I did a lot of soul searching, which led to defining a clearer boundary between the therapy work being done under Water & Stone and everything else I was developing or offering. This led to the founding of Firefly & Phoenix LLC, the sister company to Water & Stone. Having two separate companies with different missions has clarified a lot of what I hope to do in the future. For now, Firefly & Phoenix gives me opportunities to focus on supporting other therapists in changing the world.

Plans are underway to start an online school for people who want to go into private practice and for therapists to enjoy affordable continuing education workshops. I want to expand the annual conference I run for therapists, so more people will have access. Along those lines, I hope to offer more weekend opportunities for those who work during the week, and hold occasional two- or three-day retreats that focus on everything from dealing with burnout or anxiety to bringing creativity into your everyday life.

On the Water & Stone side, we are rebuilding and expanding once again with a couple of new therapists and my wonderful virtual assistant. Eventually, I would love to have a new in-person office or studio space that supports creativity and therapy. Our traveling to organizations was brought to a standstill during the pandemic, so I am excited to rebuild in new and sustainable ways over the next couple of years.

In the end, I hope to impact not only the communities around me but to also create a ripple effect through all the people I mentor, teach, and support. Seeing the ripples carry into new corners of the world and watching people I have supported inspire others is an indescribable experience. I cannot wait to see what lies ahead!

Chapter 11

# Groundswell

## The Art of Social Enterprise

*Pamela Whitaker*

### CULTIVATING NEW GROUND: THE NATURE OF SOCIAL ENTERPRISE

Groundswell combines organic, biodiversity, and climate change gardening for communities in partnership with local and national government organizations. It was developed as a service to people seeking the skills necessary to develop their own food gardens for sustainability and as an opportunity to enhance their wellness and quality of life. The founding aim of Groundswell was to incorporate art therapy with the art of organic gardening to contribute to not only domestic food cultivation but also the development of human nature and the environmental supports necessary for health and enhanced life satisfaction in rural areas.

Located near the border with Northern Ireland (in County Louth), Groundswell is situated in a rural peninsula, approximately halfway between Belfast and Dublin. As a rural development initiative, it received start-up funding from Ireland's National Development Plan in 2006 to support social enterprise in rural regions. As part of this plan, the Leader (2020) initiative was developed to encourage community-led projects which promoted enterprise thinking (to improve the lives of people), social inclusion, and enhancements to the rural environment. The key principles of the Leader program are regional local development, networking, innovation, and cooperation, which encourage a widening perspective regarding rural localities implementing the skills necessary for community-led strategies.

A social enterprise is a business dedicated to enhancing the lives of people and achieving beneficial social, societal, and environmental impacts (Government of Ireland, 2024). The primary partners of Groundswell are

DOI: 10.4324/9781032615776-12

local governmental departments responsible for environmental, arts, and heritage services and national government agencies dedicated to rural development. In recent years, Creative Ireland has been a pivotal partner, with its national ambition to inspire and transform people, places, and communities through creativity (Creative Ireland, 2024). Creative Ireland is "committed to the vision that every person in Ireland should have the opportunity to realise their full creative potential" (Creative Ireland, 2024). Recently, Creative Ireland extended its remit to include climate action, and Groundswell is contributing arts-based research services that enhance public education in relation to climate change gardening as part of the Louth Urban Food Sanctuary project (www.louthurbanfoodsanctuary.com). As the effects of climate change in Ireland include an increased frequency of rainstorms (with flooding and strong winds), the current food-growing methods will no longer be viable. For example, edible plants cultivated in rows will be vulnerable to changing weather conditions, which will cause plants to wilt and drown. Climate-mitigating growing designs, such as edible meadows and food forests with an entanglement of edible species growing together, are an example of regenerative food growing embracing biodiversity.

Growing food contributes to the circular economy, which involves the sharing of resources and reusing assets that are already freely available as possessions or by way of civic access. This is a strengths-based model of health, which encourages gardening as a cultural activity that positively impacts both the environment and quality of life. Enterprise thinking responds to changing situations through problem-solving and teamwork. Groundswell has teamed with climate and biodiversity officers and Creative Ireland to develop public education workshops for networks of community growers seeking regenerative growing strategies. Gardening contributes to mental health, with evidence indicating that it reduces anxiety and stress levels while enhancing mood and contributing to feelings of pride and belonging (Thompson, 2018). There is also an association to self-efficacy, the execution of goal achievement, and the performance of skills which produce a sense of accomplishment. The vision of Groundswell is to deliver environmental education for people of all ages, as a psychosocial service contributing to life-long learning, social interaction, and belonging (Borgaonkar, 2023). This is also a vision that encourages changemaking, active citizenship, and the capacity to re-make our surroundings. Flourishing, a feature of positive psychology, corresponds to meaning, purpose, optimism, and acts of agency (Logan et al., 2023). Generative acts (such as gardening) enhance the neuropsychology of flourishing (Kong et al., 2020). As a physical activity, gardening encourages attention restoration and contributes toward neuroplasticity, activating core brain networks that strengthen cognitive functions (Lentoor, 2024). Gardening also supports executive functions related to flexible thinking, impulse control, working memory, planning and prioritizing, initiation, and organization (Lentoor, 2024).

The vision of Groundswell is to enhance quality-of-life indicators in partnership with government and education services. Quality of life in rural areas has been characterized by education and knowledge generation, landscape and cultural heritage, health security, environment, and well-being (Beltramo et al., 2024). The current National Development Plan of Ireland (2021–2030) recognizes the significance of local improvement schemes, rural regeneration, and community enhancement as contributors to life satisfaction. Resilience within rural areas is linked to culture, the arts, and social cohesion. The environment brings people together as a shared resource which becomes a strategic foundation upon which to co-produce growth. Investment in rural heritage protects and allies with nature, allowing people to come together and participate in the shared resources of the landscape commons (Government of Ireland, 2021). The commons is a shared community landscape which promotes democratic decision-making, the sharing of knowledge and skills, cooperative food growing, and the gifting of materials and labor. Ponstingel (2023) has researched the impact of community food gardens within the diverse economies framework, particularly their contribution to food security, social capital, civic greening, health, and community identity—all contributing to the production of place. Environmental education empowers community growers "to share seeds, to share harvests, to share recipes, to share knowledge, to use common resources (e.g., water) and to perform duties like composting and recycling" (Ponstingel, 2023, p. 2). As a representation of reciprocity, a community garden represents transactions outside of the market economy, particularly in relation to shared exchanges that offer material sustenance (Community Partnering for Local Development, n.d.).

Shared decision-making can influence new ideas that manifest in cooperative enterprise. Community gardens offer an opportunity to produce food security through shared cultivation and harvest. Groundswell encourages open-source food and biodiversity landscaping that expresses divergency, as an alternative to the homogenization of public spaces (produced by omnipresent and non-aligned landscape designs), which can be subject to public indifference and disengagement (Biesta, 2012; Kellhammer, 2008) (Figure 11.1). Open-source landscaping relinquishes horticultural control and encourages people to be influenced by nature as an artistic experience. It also adopts the use of plants as graffiti in the form of improvisational guerrilla gardening. The inspiration for food availability, in the thoroughfares of everyday life, also references the following food activists acting as agents for landscape liberation: Oliver Kellhammer's botanical

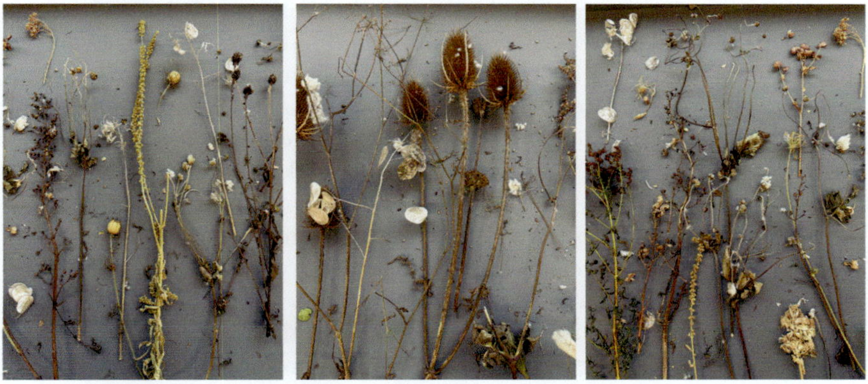

*Figure 11.1* *Rewilding: Wild plants harvested in the Groundswell garden for community seed sharing at the Void Arts Centre (Northern Ireland). These medicinal and wildflower specimens are botanical interventions promoting naturescapes in civic life.*

interventions for community sustenance and repair (Kellhammer, 2008); Ron Finley's gardening *gangsta* project in Los Angeles (encouraging rebellious and ubiquitous food planting in public landscapes) (Finley, 2024); Richard Reynolds and the UK guerrilla gardening manifesto (Reynolds, 2024); and the Incredible Edible civic food landscapes in Todmorden, Yorkshire (Incredible Edible, 2024).

## AN ETHOS OF HOSPITALITY

Groundswell's vision has always included an ethos of hospitality, originally inspired by the writings of Gilles Deleuze and Félix Guattari (2004) and their use of the botanical term "rhizome" to describe growth in multiple directions (or simultaneous growth in the commons). A rhizome is an assemblage of life and a system of aggregate growth, which exists as an expanding network; it describes an ecology of people and territories of potential (Whitaker, 2012). This is a recognition of land potentials that may be unrecognized or lying dormant, ready to be cultivated. The community landscape invites us in, so that we can grow. Home and neighborhood are linked through gardening that also initiates spontaneous cultural practices whereby people feel comfortable in the places around them (de Certeau, 1998). The public homeplace is an extension of home, in the routines of everyday life (Timm-Bottos, 2005). It receives people's desire to be given to by their locality, in terms of feeling represented in its composition and attributes. This is not a reference to commercial hospitality, but hospitality as a collective resourcing of assets. Everyone brings something to the community landscape as offerings of themselves and their nature (what they want to grow), including their vision for changing the world around them. The community table model within art therapy is an example of collaborative helping and how each person has something distinct to offer within social and political commentaries around a shared space (Lloyd & Usiskin, 2022). “In a world marked by division, the land of hospitality serves as a beacon of hope, showing us that we can embrace our differences and find unity in our shared humanity” (Medium, 2023).

Hospitality is an expression of humanity's shared existence and mutual trust, and it expresses a relationship of generosity (RTE, 2024). Gardening is inherently giving in relation to sharing, seeds, plants, and produce. There is also the sharing of horticultural skills, gardening tools, local land, meals, recipes, and celebrations of the growing seasons. Groundswell acts as a curator of potential. The goal is to be partners in production and bring everyone to a community table by way of the expertise of everyone's lived experience. This is also the creation of comfort, making people feel at home in their surroundings and encouraging them to share their cultures of gardening as expressions of their identity and communion with nature. A series of gardens is a public art installation and gardeners are artists producing habitats contributing to a greater environmental assemblage. We can give to others through offering what we have made as a gesture of conviviality which can influence “attitudes, preferences and behavioural intentions” (Godovykh, 2024). The art of gardening is a creative act, assembling living art media into a composition. The immersive appeal of gardens can create an atmosphere of welcome which also engages with a viewer's symbolic associations and emotional responses (Godovykh, 2024). Hospitality generates an impression and acknowledges guests as companions in an experience, which is key to a social enterprise supporting inclusion and participation.

## ART THERAPY PEDAGOGY: CAREER PORTFOLIOS

Groundswell has contributed to higher education teaching by developing cultural practicums as part of students' practice-based learning at the Belfast School of Art. These social enterprise projects offer professional skills associated with the creative industries. Art therapy could also be considered a creative industry that contributes to life quality through the design of services on a community to clinical continuum. Cultural practicums are project-based opportunities to develop skills in proposal writing, project management, design thinking, visual communication, teamwork, and program delivery. Students are encouraged to develop their professional portfolios through project practicums where they can develop both leadership and curation skills. Service design is a key feature of cultural practicums which encourages students to propose the planning of a new service in conjunction with experts with lived experience (clients or service users) who are partners within public health, education, social care, or therapeutic services. Typically, art therapy training includes employability skills for careers within singular organizations; however, in reality, art therapists have portfolio careers which combine multiple contracts with several art therapy service providers. Entrepreneurial skills are essential to develop a portfolio showcasing a flexible and responsive approach to art therapy delivery, which aligns with the strategies and vision of each employer. It is also important to align art therapy with the specific mission of each organization and to consider government strategies and policies that inform the funding of art therapy services. Financial support is linked to art therapy's social impact which influences participants' life quality and standards of living. This knowledge assists art therapists in defining how to compose a project or service that delivers impact on a larger scale connecting therapeutic services with social agendas.

Nolan (2024) and Timm-Bottos (2017) describe the significance of community and public practice art therapy as forms of activism which incorporate mutuality and co-design. This is art therapy which facilitates shared leadership amongst all participants and encourages mentoring and purpose (Kaimal et al., 2017). Facilitative leadership envisions a creative and just future amongst participants who use their talents and abilities to expand the scope of art therapy into a bigger picture awareness of civic society (Kaimal et al., 2017). This is also about anticipating the future of the profession and its potential contributions to social policies and strategic development on a community, regional, and national scale. Timm-Bottos refers to "enabling spaces" (places apart from home and work) as places where art therapists can work at the front lines of where people gather. "We are beginning to see how art therapists have the potential to mobilise large numbers of people across sociopolitical divides" (Timm-Bottos, 2017, p. 96). The accessibility of these third spaces, as civic comfort zones, can be locations where innovation in art therapy can be nurtured from emergent knowledges developed within participatory places (Backos & Carolan, 2017). Timm-Bottos founded the Art Hive movement (open studios within civic society) as a site of training and engaged scholarship for art therapy trainees at Concordia University (Montreal). Art Hive studios welcome everyone as an artist with free access to art materials and psychological supports (Art Hives, 2024). The regenerative ethos of the Art Hive movement has become an international movement with local studios being supported in libraries, arts and cultural centers, gardens, and neighborhoods around the world.

Groundswell has contributed to environmental art therapy practice, public practice art therapy, and festival art therapy, which consider art therapy as an expression of civic engagement. Innovations in art therapy practice can be composed within third spaces which de-colonize the authority of the art therapist, and art therapy pedagogies, rooted in individualized psychological and developmental theories. Third space offers the potential for the commons to evoke the sharing of space, skills, and information. Keng (2024) endorses community actualization over self-actualization, arguing that art therapy education is often conditioned by theoretical imperialism, which imposes limitations upon the stories of human experience composed within the landscapes of daily living as "heterogeneous multiplicities and multidimensional subjectivity" (Keng, 2024, p. 10).

Social enterprise in the creative sector should lead art therapists to an appreciation of how to influence collective actions. Beyond individual and group art therapy there is the potential of developing social movements where participants are creating new life potentials based on their lived experience expertise. Social capital is the capacity to build networks to promote the common good, to bond together as enterprising citizens and to make something happen that has social benefit for daily life (Dimitrova, 2023). Promoting cooperation with others challenges neo-liberal associations to enterprise being aligned to market forces which can be detrimental to health and social well-being. Within neo-liberalism, competition and self-interest are valued over the attributes of cooperation and the sharing of resources. An emphasis on individualism can contribute to loneliness and mistrust (Card & Hepburn, 2023). Developing environments for health promotion challenges the role of psychological theories which *responsibalize* the individual to manage their own mental health (Card & Hepburn, 2023). Fancourt et al. (2022) describe wellness as getting the most from our lives and reaching our potential. Finding meaning and purpose through social activations and environmental curation encourages capacity and nurturing a purposeful identity evolving with positive social relations and the ecologies of life (Fancourt et al., 2022).

Wood and McKoy-Lewens comment that it is "strange how the effects of social and health inequalities are rarely acknowledged within . . . art therapy . . . because the focus of therapy has tended to stay on the inner world" (Wood & McKoy-Lewens, 2023, p. 28). It is important to acknowledge the ways in which art therapy education has not identified the socio-political realities of service users who have lived experience of being othered and excluded (Wood & McKoy-Lewens, 2023). Eastwood et al. (2023) call for the embedding of anti-oppressive practice within art therapy education, which considers the impacts of power, inequality, and discrimination. This is why civic, environmental, and cultural art therapy practices need to be understood as a social enterprise which promotes agency and visibility. Public practice and social justice art therapy models promote agency that mediates between individual, relational, and communal goals as a curation of artistic activism (Potash & Kalmanowitz, 2023). Social enterprise takes people outdoors and into places where they can activate through their aggregate intentions. The civic studio is a place for imagining solutions and focusing upon transformative collective leadership (Potash & Kalmanowitz, 2023). Collective leadership has been identified as an approach to healthcare that co-designs interventions, for the purpose of inclusivity and ethical outcomes. It is an attribute of social enterprise, as it involves everyone's talents and skills to implement a place-based ethic of care, changing the nature of everyday places into expressions of public artistry (Bird, 2023; De Brún et al., 2019; Goralnik et al., 2014). Social enterprise art therapy should create the conditions for participatory democracy and knowledge making which challenges dominant narratives regarding land use, thereby liberating people to become the influencers of their own public homeplaces as environmental citizens.

## IMPLICATIONS: REBRANDING ART THERAPY

This chapter proposes the practice of social enterprise art therapy as both a strategy of collective activism and training for art therapists within higher education. It has emphasized the imperative of art therapists to align with national and local governmental development plans, which produce funding opportunities for art therapists in regard to health promotion and quality of life outcomes. This is an opportunity for art therapy to extend its vision outwards and to create the conditions for public practice, with the goal of cultivating environments as life studios. People should be nurtured to become artists in residence in their own public homeplaces. As a creative industry, art therapy can encourage emergent knowledge and skills which are familiar to art and design students, but may be deficient within art therapy training. Whereas art therapy trainees are proficient in clinical and research skills, their potential as social entrepreneurs should also encompass leadership and innovation, which are the foundations for a socially responsive career portfolio. Innovations in art therapy are not solely derived from clinical practice, but are also composed from public projects with community stakeholders. The "shared creation of knowledge in art therapy and the valuing of community wisdom allows the profession to grow and strengthen its knowledge base" (Backos & Carolan, 2017, p. 52). The production of the community table, third spaces, the public homeplace, and environmental stewardship are all attributes of social enterprise that can imagine something more for the profession of art therapy. Environmental scholar

Donna Haraway's concept of *natureculture* describes the entanglement of humans with their ecologies, which is a social enterprise of kinship that recognizes that our existence happens within an ecology of life supports (Keng, 2024). Art therapy has the potential to "re-enchant the disenchanted familiar" (Keng, 2024, p. 239) through activating artistry as a duty of care to people, place and potentials. Life configures beings (the human and the more than human) within everyday practices that need care and attention and empathetic actions of solidarity. Enterprise art therapy, in the context of this chapter, is the courage to make nature happen within both domestic and civic homeplaces as a chance for not only place-based recovery but also for the enhancement of all existence.

## REFERENCES

Art Hives. (2024). *What is the art hive network?* Retrieved from https://arthives.org/about

Backos, A., & Carolan, R. (2017). Art therapy pedagogy. In R. Carolan & A. Backos (Eds.), *Emerging perspectives in art therapy: Trends, movements and developments* (pp. 48–57). Routledge.

Beltramo, R., Peira, G., Pasino, G., & Bonadonna, A. (2024). Quality of life in rural areas: A set of indicators for improving wellbeing. *Sustainability, 16*(5), 1804. Retrieved from www.mdpi.com/2071–1050/16/5/1804

Biesta, G. (2012). Becoming public: Public pedagogy, citizenship and the public sphere. *Social and Cultural Geography, 13*(7), 683–697.

Bird, J. (2023). *Social action art therapy in a time of crisis.* Routledge.

Borgaonkar, C. (2023, July 31). The mental health continuum: Flourishing, languishing and everything in between. *Public Health Insight, 43*(2), 207–222. Retrieved from https://thepublichealthinsight.com/the-mental-health-continuum-flourishing-languishing-and-everything-in-between/

Card, K., & Hepburn, K. (2023). Is neoliberalism killing us? A cross sectional study of the impact of neoliberalism on health and social wellbeing in the midst of the COVID-19 pandemic. *International Journal of Social Determinants of Health and Health Services, 53*(3), 363–373.

Community Partnering for Local Development. (n.d.). *Diverse economies framework.* Retrieved from www.communitypartnering.info

Creative Ireland. (2024). *About us.* Retrieved from www.creativeireland.gov.ie/en/about/

De Brún, A., O'Donovan, R., & McAuliffe, E. (2019). Interventions to develop collectivistic leadership in healthcare settings: A systematic review. *BMC Health Services Research, 19*(1), 72. Retrieved from https://bmchealthservres.biomedcentral.com/articles/10.1186/s12913-019-3883-x

De Certeau, M. (1998). The neighborhood. In M. De Certeau, L. Giard, & P. Mayol (Eds.), *The practice of everyday life: Volume 2 living and cooking* (pp. 7–15). University of Minnesota Press.

Deleuze, G., & Guattari, F. (2004). *A thousand plateaus*. Continuum.

Dimitrova, M. (2023). *Social entrepreneurship in the creative industries*. WASP Foundation.

Eastwood, C., McDonald, A., Turner, D., & Vernon OBE, P. (2023). Intersectionality and art therapy. *International Journal of Art Therapy, 28*(1–2), 2–6.

Fancourt, D., Bone, J. K., Bu, F., Mak, H. W., & Bradbury, A. (2022). *The impact of arts and cultural engagement on population health*. University College London. Retrieved from https://sbbresearch.org/wp-content/uploads/2023/03/Arts-and-population-health-FINAL-March-2023.pdf

Finley, R. (2024). *The Ron Finley project*. Retrieved from www.ronfinley.com

Godovykh, M. (2024). Hospitality art experience model: The effects of visual art on guests' attitudes and behavior. *Tourism and Hospitality, 5*(2), 439–447.

Goralnik, L., Dobson, T., & Nelson, M. P. (2014). Place-based care ethics: A field philosophy pedagogy. *Canadian Journal of Environmental Education, 19*(2024), 180–196. Retrieved from https://cjee.lakeheadu.ca/article/view/1279

Government of Ireland, Department of Public Expenditure and Reform. (2021). *National development plan: 2021–2030*. Retrieved from www.gov.ie/en/publication/774e2-national-development-plan-2021–2030/

Government of Ireland, Department of Rural and Community Development. (2024). *Social enterprise*. Retrieved from www.gov.ie/en/publication/624c74-social-enterprise/

Incredible Edible. (2024). *We are incredible edible todmorden*. Retrieved from https://incredible-edible-todmorden.co.uk

Kaimal, G., Metzl, E., & Millrod, E. (2017). Facilitative leadership: A framework for the creative arts therapies. *Art Therapy: Journal of the American Art Therapy Association, 34*(3), 146–151.

Kellhammer, O. (2008). *Botanical interventions: Open source landscape and community repair*. Retrieved from www.oliverk.org/publications/non-fiction/botanical-interventions-open-source-landscape-and-community-repair-essay

Keng, E. S. Y. (2024). *Exploring the third space borderland in art therapy education and practice* [Doctoral dissertation]. Charles Darwin University. Retrieved from https://ris.cdu.edu.au/ws/portalfiles/portal/94673103/Thesis_CDU_San_E.pdf

Kong, F., Heller, A. S., van Reekum, C. M., & Sato, W. (2020). Positive neuroscience: The neuroscience of human flourishing. *Frontiers in Human Neuroscience, 14*(47), 1–3.

Leader. (2020). *About the leader programme*. Retrieved from https://nationalrural-network.ie/leader/

Lentoor, A. G. (2024). Effect of gardening physical activity on neuroplasticity and cognitive function. *Exploration of Neuroprotective Therapy, 2024*(4), 251–272.

Lloyd, B., & Usiskin, M. (2022). The community table: Developing art therapy studios on, in-between, and across borders. In C. Brown & H. Omand (Eds.), *Contemporary practice in studio art therapy* (pp. 101–117). Routledge.

Logan, A. C., Berman, B. M., & Prescott, S. L. (2023). Vitality revisited: The evolving concept of flourishing and its relevance to personal and public health. *International Journal of Environmental Research and Public Health, 20*(6), 5065.

Medium. (2023). *The land of hospitality: A journey of heartwarming experiences.* Retrieved from https://medium.com/@iramnadeem2434/the-land-of-hospitality-a-journey-of-heartwarming-experiences-3746df5b8c5a

Nolan, E. G. (2024). *Community art therapy.* Routledge.

Ponstingel, D. (2023). Community gardens as commons through the lens of the diverse economies framework. *Applied Geography, 154*(6), 102945.

Potash, J., & Kalmanowitz, D. (2023). Art therapists as activists in social movements. *Journal of Peacebuilding and Development, 18*(3), 310–328.

Reynolds, R. (2024). *Guerrilla gardening.* Retrieved from www.guerrillagardening.org/index.html

RTE. (2024). *How to soften corners: Jennie Moran's philosophy of hospitality.* Retrieved from www.rte.ie/culture/2024/0427/1445027-how-to-soften-corners-jennie-morans-philosophy-of-hospitality/

Thompson, R. (2018). Gardening for health: A regular dose of gardening. *Clinical Medicine, 18*(3), 201–205.

Timm-Bottos, J. (2005). *The necessity of public homeplace in urban revitalisation* [Doctoral dissertation]. The University of New Mexico. Retrieved from www.proquest.com/openview/a1fa08201ab4b3b2e543cc8e8a5897de/1?pq-origsite=gscholar&cbl=18750&diss=y

Timm-Bottos, J. (2017). Public practice art therapy: Enabling spaces across North America. *Canadian Art Therapy Association Journal, 30*(2), 94–99.

Whitaker, P. (2012). The art therapy assemblage. In H. Burt (Ed.), *Art therapy and postmodernism: Creative healing through a prism* (pp. 344–367). Jessica Kingsley.

Wood, C., & McKoy-Lewens, J. (2023). An art therapy education response: Linking inequality and intersectional identity. *International Journal of Art Therapy, 28*(1–2), 28–37.

# Conclusion
# Driving Change

## Embracing the Limitless Potential of Our Creative Resources

*Jennifer Marie DeLucia*

In a 2011 guest editorial for *Art Therapy: Journal of the American Art Therapy Association,* Pat Allen challenged readers to consider our role as art therapists outside of the clinical setting, and beyond the studio. Citing Cliff Joseph (1997), she declared that we are obligated to a larger social responsibility and must acknowledge the interconnectedness between what is good for art therapy and what is good for our clients, our colleagues, the earth and all its inhabitants. As the field embraces expansive ways of conceptualizing our practice beyond the clinic and studio, as Allen suggests, we can leverage our relational, creative, and entrepreneurial potential to promote innovation and change.

In curating this edited book, my goal has been to broaden the ways art therapists conceptualize their work in communities. By introducing social entrepreneurship and highlighting examples of art therapists promoting social change, I have aimed to inspire and guide future efforts. For instance, in Chapter 2 ("Culture Circle Studios: Unifying a School Community in Healthy Relationships"), Emily Goldstein Nolan describes the evolution of a program designed to build healthy relationship skills among educators. The program started with a small group of educators, gained buy-in from the school community, and over time expanded to a district-wide program and subsequently a task-sharing model with a published facilitator's manual. The program was structured to respond to the evolving needs of the participants, and several key partners within the school setting were involved in the initial phases of the project, ultimately creating the conditions for its success.

The field of social entrepreneurship is rich with related work that can serve as a source of inspiration and guidance as art therapists continue to

DOI: 10.4324/9781032615776-13

tackle issues affecting the communities we serve. By adopting entrepreneurial approaches, art therapists can develop solutions that are sustainable and impactful. For example, in Chapter 11 ("Groundswell: The Art of Social Enterprise"), Pamela Whitaker describes a social enterprise in Ireland that partnered with local and national government organizations to support domestic food cultivation and enhance quality of life and personal well-being by incorporating art therapy with the art of organic gardening. She explains how Groundswell acts as a "curator of potential," with community partnering in production and sharing expertise from their unique lived experiences. Likewise, in Chapter 4 ("The Living Museum, a Contemporary Art Movement"), Mitra Reyhani Ghadim and Rose Ehemann describe how, in 1983, a 40,000-square-foot abandoned psychiatric building in New York City was transformed into a space where everyone was welcomed as an artist and creativity flourished—the first Living Museum. Over the last 20 years, Reyhani and Ehemann have supported the development of Living Museums internationally, noting how the model is sustainable because of its adaptable design, which can be tailored to various settings. Both examples demonstrate how sustainability was addressed through strategic partnerships, flexible design, innovative use of resources, and community engagement.

Social entrepreneurship provides a lens to view grassroots community-based efforts, and national and global initiatives in art therapy that address social issues, aligning with our ethics and guiding values of beneficence and justice. Our ethical principles describe our responsibility to engage in activities that serve the betterment of society. In Chapter 8, authors Jessica Woolhiser Stallings, Jenelle Miller, Yasmin Henderson, and Jennifer Jividen Jackson addressed the need for enforceable standards of practice in the state of Nebraska to protect the public from potential harm. There are many forms social entrepreneurship in art therapy can take, from advocacy to promote policy change as demonstrated in Chapter 8 ("Social Entrepreneurship in Licensure and Educational Advocacy"), creating accessible art therapy training programs as described in Chapter 9 ("Academic Program Development as Social Entrepreneurship"), and tailoring services to the needs of historically marginalized groups as illustrated in Chapter 5 ("Healing Work is Justice Work: The Development and Marketing of Art Therapy Services Using an Intersectionality Framework"). Applying the framework of social entrepreneurship enables us to identify specific skills we can reinforce in art therapy training, supervision, practice, and mentorship. Promoting the advancement of entrepreneurial skills builds on related experience and knowledge that art therapists have developed through their education and professional practice and will support them to engage in social entrepreneurship.

Art therapists are adept at assessment and often have unique ground-level perspectives on community issues and needs, which grow out of their day-to-day practice with individuals, couples, families, and communities. For example, in Chapter 6 ("Creating a Self-Contained Mobile Art Therapy Facility"), Lisa Lonsbury discussed how the idea for a mobile art therapy studio emerged from her work in the community. She identified challenges with physical space and access to services while providing art therapy on a contractual basis which inspired her to develop a solution. Direct knowledge of community issues helps art therapists understand the needs and concerns of the communities they serve. In addition, they have the skills and experience necessary to coordinate community participation. For example, in Chapter 3 ("Art Activism for Social Change"), Mary Andrus discusses Art for Social Change, an art activism group formed in a higher education setting. Andrus and the group's co-founder invited partners across campus to participate, and group members initiated a two-year participatory action research cycle. The resulting reflection, dialogue, and action resulted in a shared leadership structure, vision, and reflexive structure that valued the participation of all members.

Observing the role of art therapists within their communities reveals that many are already employing social entrepreneurial skills in their daily practice. A recent survey found that art therapists frequently use entrepreneurial skills such as vision and goal-setting, resource management, strategic communication, measuring outcomes, and creating innovative solutions (DeLucia & Linsner, 2025). Despite using these skills regularly, most art therapists reported having no formal training in them (DeLucia & Linsner, 2025). Survey participants did note a strong overlap between their practice and training as art therapists and the skills needed for successful engagement in social entrepreneurship. For example, in Chapter 10 ("The Ripple Effect of Entrepreneurship: Increasing Impact Through Evolution"), Emery Hurst Mikel discusses how she leveraged her experience as an artist and former theatre director to develop a successful business model addressing the need for increased access to services for older adults. Noting that she was not able to locate any related literature in the field of art therapy, she relied on business literature, mentorship, and her own creativity to guide the way. Inspired by such examples, future research in this area may explore art therapists' effectiveness with these skills and their training preferences, to best align their identified needs with the curriculum and training in graduate programs, art therapy supervision, mentorship, and professional development opportunities (DeLucia & Linsner, 2025).

Art therapists may identify issues, champion processes to address them, or coordinate resources to mobilize others. Many art therapists may not recognize their potential as social entrepreneurs or view their work as entrepreneurial. They may start with limited confidence, questioning their understanding of an issue and their opportunities to act. Social issues often have deeply embedded roots, and it can be daunting to consider how to untangle and address these issues. It is helpful to remember that this work is best accomplished when done in collaboration with others. This benefit is highlighted in Chapter 7 ("Queer Coalition Building in the Creative Arts Therapies: A Personal Reflection and Introduction"), where Zachary D. Van Den Berg shares how attendee feedback from Expressing Pride, an online symposium featuring contemporary practice and research in LGBTQIA+ affirmative care, illuminated the benefits of a distributed approach to leadership. The resulting organizational shift supported sustainability and expansion of Expressive Pride and the Coalition for Queer Creative Arts Therapies.

The initiatives presented in this book illustrate the essential role social entrepreneurship plays in art therapy. The grassroots efforts described in each chapter emerged from a ground-level view of the issues and served to promote change, address unmet needs, and provide a sense of stability, community, and hope. Social entrepreneurial art therapists foster these initiatives by actively listening to and responding to constituent communities. Their ventures not only serve the community but also leverage its support, sustaining initiatives through widespread buy-in and participation. Community participation enhances the effectiveness of initiatives by ensuring they are relevant to the people they serve.

Recognizing the importance of these efforts, educators, supervisors, and mentors must provide training and mentorship on the skills associated with successful entrepreneurship, like managing resources, vision, and goal-setting; engaging key partners; creating innovative solutions; measuring outcomes; mobilizing existing resources; and strategic communication. As discussed in Chapter 1 ("Creative Changemaker: Art Therapist as Social Entrepreneur"), many of these entrepreneurial skills parallel art therapists' existing knowledge and experience. However, additional training and mentorship may support art therapists in advancing these skills to address broader challenges related to systems, policies, and social issues. Training and mentorship may be particularly valuable at the graduate level or during entry into the field, as it will help new practitioners to envision the interconnectedness of their work with the broader needs of society.

I have experienced the generosity of leaders in our field who routinely share their time and expertise by serving as mentors and offering their support and encouragement to others in the field. A love of the profession and a desire to advance the field and practice of art therapy are at the heart of these efforts. Training and mentorship can help newer practitioners envision the interconnectedness of their work with the broader needs of society. As we continue to evolve the field, let us all embody the generosity of our leaders and embrace the limitless potential of our creative resources to drive social change.

## REFERENCES

Allen, P. B. (2011). Special issue on the social action and advocacy paradigm in art therapy: The lens of art therapy opens larger still. *Art Therapy: Journal of the American Art Therapy Association, 28*(2), 48–49. https://doi.org/10.1080/07421656.2011.579892

DeLucia, J. M., & Linsner, R. K. (2025). Creating impactful change: An exploration of art therapists' experiences related to entrepreneurship. *Art Therapy: Journal of the American Art Therapy Association,* 1–13.

Joseph, C. (1997). Reflections on the inescapable political dimensions of art and live. In P. M. Farris-Dufrene (Ed.), *Voices of color: Art and society in the Americas* (pp. 46–54). Humanities Press International.

# Index

*Note*: Page numbers in *italics* indicate figures, and page numbers in **bold** indicate tables in the text.

For Product Safety Concerns and Information please contact our EU representative GPSR@taylorandfrancis.com Taylor & Francis Verlag GmbH, Kaufingerstraße 24, 80331 München, Germany